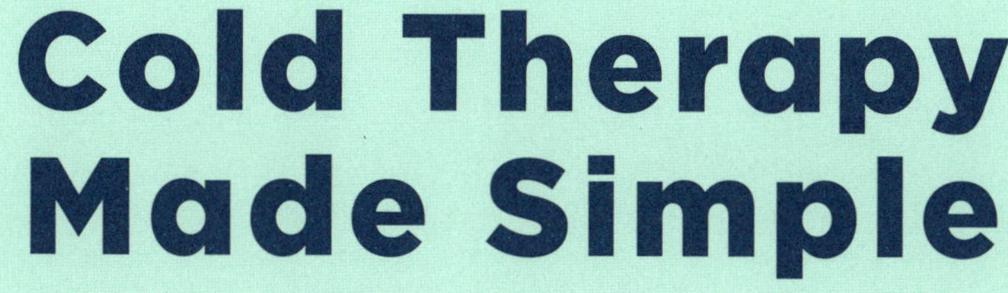

Cold Therapy Made Simple

A 5-Step Guide to Using Cold Exposure to Heal Better, Recover Faster, and Live Longer

Chris Peterson

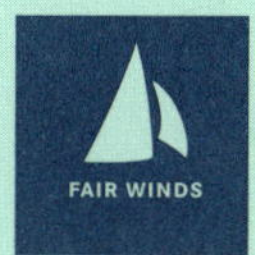

Quarto.com

First Published in 2026 by Fair Winds Press, an imprint of The Quarto Group, 100 Cummings Center, Suite 265-D, Beverly, MA 01915, USA.
T (978) 282-9590 F (978) 283-2742

EEA Representation, WTS Tax d.o.o., Žanova ulica 3, 4000 Kranj, Slovenia. www.wts-tax.si

Fair Winds Press titles are also available at discount for retail, wholesale, promotional, and bulk purchase. For details, contact the Special Sales Manager by email at specialsales@quarto.com or by mail at The Quarto Group, Attn: Special Sales Manager, 100 Cummings Center, Suite 265-D, Beverly, MA 01915, USA.

30 29 28 27 26 1 2 3 4 5

ISBN: 978-1-57715-684-0

Digital edition published in 2026
eISBN: 978-1-57715-685-7

Library of Congress Cataloging-in-Publication Data is available.

Design and Page Layout: Laura Shaw
Illustration: Studio Quarante Douze, Emmanuelle Desfossés, www.quarantedouze.ca

The content on pages 108–109 previously appeared in *The Power of Breathwork* (Fair Winds Press 2020) by Jennifer Patterson. The content on pages 112–116 previously appeared in *The Power of Guided Meditation* (Fair Winds Press 2021) by Jessica Crow.

Printed in Guangdong, China TT122025

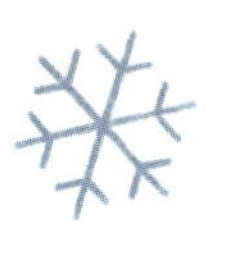
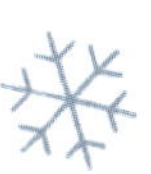

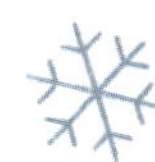
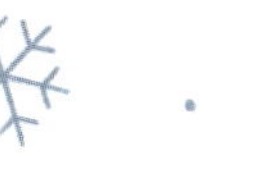
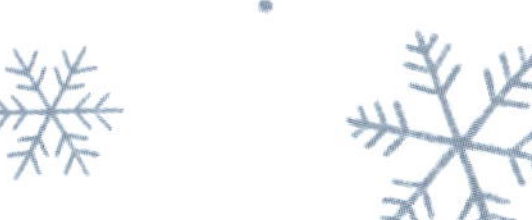
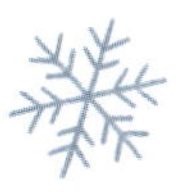
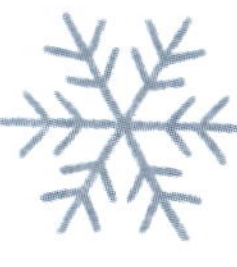
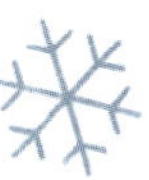

I dedicate this book to all those
seeking better health and wellness with
simple life practices and lifestyle changes.
I hope this is a powerful tool in
your healthspan journey.

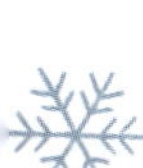
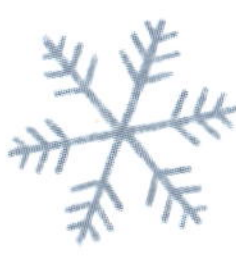
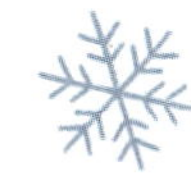
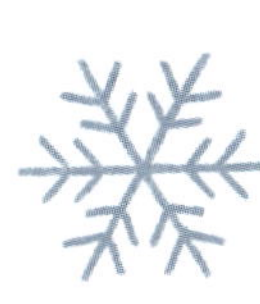
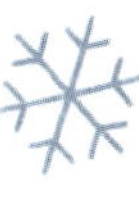
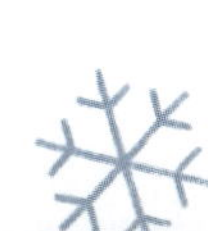
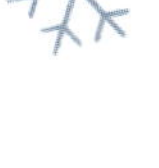
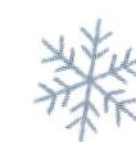
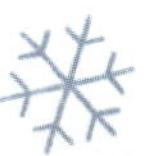
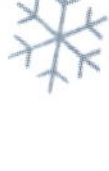

CONTENTS

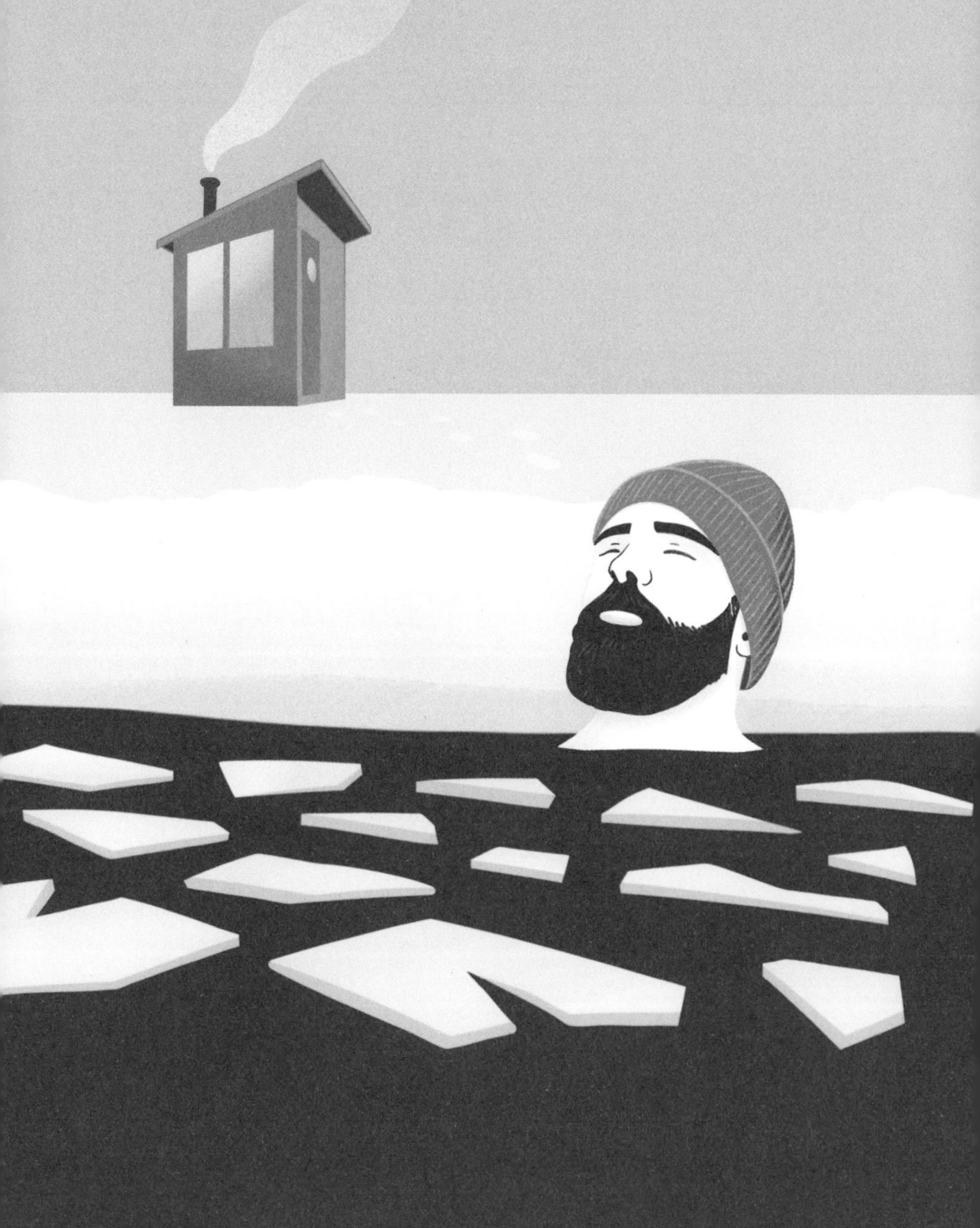

INTRODUCTION

We humans don't like to be cold and uncomfortable. From the moment our cave-dwelling ancestors sparked the first fire, we've associated warmth with security and contentment. But, as it turns out, this has a downside. Our understandable embrace of comfort may have prevented us from exploring a potentially valuable—and maybe even transformative—health and wellness resource: the power of cold.

Intentionally and regularly subjecting all or part of your body to extreme cold in a practice known as "cold therapy" is, well, not the most pleasant experience. But an increasing body of evidence points to the very real possibility that this therapy offers a whole range of health and wellness benefits. This book explores the science behind those benefits and debunks myths and misunderstandings that come along with this type of therapy. This is a data-driven investigation of the ways in which cold exposure can potentially improve your physical and mental health, and overall well-being.

Cold therapy's potential spans both treatment and prevention. It has been used to address a wide variety of diseases and conditions, from migraines to arthritis and more. Cold application can also speed recovery from injuries and reduce the trauma of surgery. Athletes and trainers long ago discovered that cold therapy can be a great tool in accelerating recovery from intense athletic exertion. There is even a good deal of evidence that cold therapy has the potential to enhance the body's immune response, and some evidence that it may slow down aging. More importantly for individuals dealing with chronic conditions, cold immersion appears to have a significant impact on pain and the inflammation that exacerbates and may even cause those disorders.

That probably sounds like a lot of tangible benefits from a treatment that appears overwhelmingly simple and a bit odd in practice. However, what seems simple in the doing relies on incredibly complex physiological and psychological processes behind the scenes. Exposing your body to extremes of cold triggers the release of many different hormones, immune-system agents, and molecular processes. In fact, there are few systems or tissues in the body that aren't impacted by cold exposure.

You may not have heard a lot about it, but cold therapy is far from a fringe idea. Even if we didn't realize it at the time, most of us have used modest cold therapy in the form of an ice pack applied to reduce swelling and pain after an injury. And medical professionals also apply cold therapy during post-operative care after many major reconstructive surgeries. As part of rotator cuff or knee replacement surgery recovery, it is standard practice to use an at-home shoulder cuff or knee ice machine for several hours each day, during which 40°F (4.4°C) water circulates around the surgical site to significantly reduce pain and recovery time.

Cold therapy is a global practice. There is a long and storied tradition throughout Scandinavia of following a session in the sauna with a quick plunge in icy waters. The contrast instantaneously sharpens your mental focus and noticeably improves mood and well-being.

Those benefits are significant, but they are just the tip of the iceberg (excuse the pun). As the concept of cold therapy has exploded in popularity, researchers have launched an ever-increasing number of studies exploring the many possible ways exposure to cold might aid health, wellness, and healing.

THE MECHANISM

Even though cold therapy is used to address many different concerns, almost all of them boil down to reducing inflammation. Inflammation is the body's natural response to injury, trauma, infection, and foreign invaders, from microbes to bullets. It's also your body's reaction to normal exertion, such as running a mile or training with weights. Inflammation is essential to healing and repairing the body, but when the reaction is too aggressive or persists, it can also be an aggravating and chronic symptom of disease and malfunction.

Basically, an inflammatory response has three objectives: nullify the cause of the trauma or condition, efficiently remove waste material (including damaged cells and tissue), and begin repairs to reverse the damage. In the normal course of our lives, inflammation helps the body stabilize injury sites and minimize pain. Specific inflammatory cells are dispersed to kill germs and get rid of toxic byproducts, among other functions.

Inflammation only becomes unhealthy when it is chronic or acute. Essentially, damage occurs when the response kicks into overdrive. For instance, in an autoimmune disease such as fibromyalgia or lupus, the inflammatory response is tricked into attacking normal healthy tissue—causing pain and damage to joints, eyes, and other susceptible structures.

One of the most effective ways to reduce inflammation is the direct application of cold. Of course, inflammation is most often an internal problem. That means cold needs to be applied strategically to have an impact. More of the body will need to be exposed, and usually at lower temperatures for a longer time. That involves some risk. Because maintaining a stable and fairly high core temperature (ideally as close to 98.6°F [37°C] as possible) is essential to the function of your organs and nervous system, there is a balance to be struck. The trick is to prevent the cold from causing more damage than it stops.

There is a distinctive right way and a wrong way to expose yourself to extreme cold temperatures. Careful adjustments are key to preventing complications and achieving exactly the positive outcome you're hoping for.

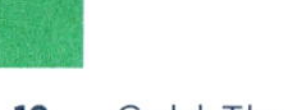

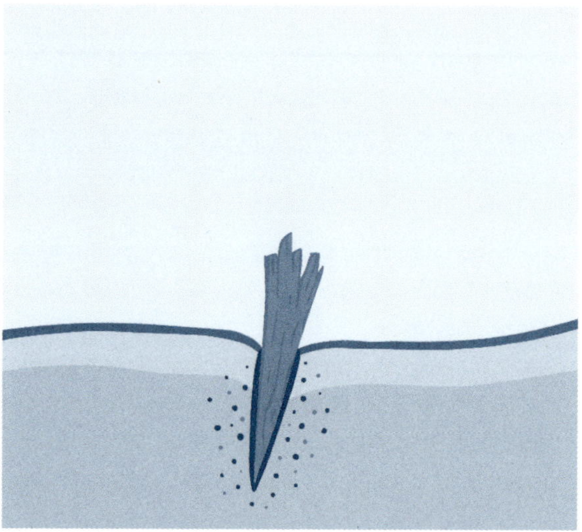

A harmful object enters the body.

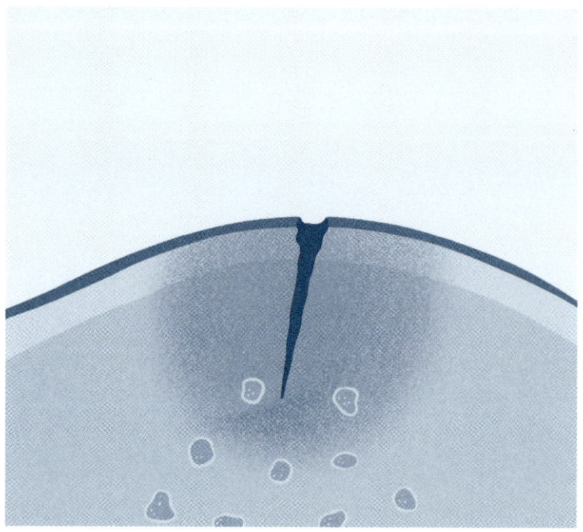

The body triggers the inflammatory response to nullify the damage and begin to repair.

THE OPTIONS

Cold can be used in many ways to address inflammation and the conditions it exacerbates. But there are several different types of cold therapy. Picking the treatment that will work best for you is a matter of deciding which technique will have the greatest impact on your particular symptoms or challenges.

The cold therapy method you choose is also a matter of personal preference. For instance, athletes have long used ice bath immersions to counter the effects of extreme exercise on muscles, tissue, and organs. Some cold therapy enthusiasts, however, prefer a more natural approach. That's led to a rising popularity in "wild swimming"—active dips in the frigid waters of lakes, rivers, or seas. In fact, there are now organizations, from international advocacy groups to local swim clubs, dedicated to this form of cold therapy. Although baths and swimming both involve immersion in low-temperature water, the process of getting in and out of the water (and what you do while you're there) differs depending on varying safety concerns and other issues.

Cold water is only one way of exposing the body to extreme low temperatures. Cold air is another. "Air chilling" can be done by simply heading outdoors on cold days wearing minimal clothing. This type of cold therapy, however, is much more precisely regulated and prone to success in a cold air "cryochamber." These structures are increasingly offered in spas and clinics. They allow for a degree of precision and control that a chilly outdoor walk or jog in a T-shirt would not.

Regardless of what type of exposure speaks to you, it's absolutely essential to consult your physician or primary caregiver before starting any cold therapy regimen. Exposure to low temperatures can pose a safety risk, particularly for anyone with a heart condition. Vascular and coronary stress are endemic to any type of cold therapy. A medical expert is best equipped to determine if the therapy you're considering might be more dangerous than helpful.

Once you're cleared for cold therapy by your health-care professional, you can start your journey into the uncomfortable world of low-temperature health and healing. Reading this book is the ideal first step.

HOW TO USE THIS BOOK

This straightforward guide is designed to hold your hand and take you step-by-step through learning about and applying cold therapy in your everyday life. In Step 1, you'll find a simple explanation of how cold works on, and in, the human body. That chapter covers both the mental and physical aspects of low-temperature exposure and, importantly, when the therapy crosses the line from beneficial to dangerous.

From there, the book will guide you through identifying your cold therapy goals, explaining the different types of cold therapy available, choosing the one that will work best for you, beginning your own practice, and refining that practice to realize the best results possible.

In the book's appendix, a resource section identifies companies that offer cold therapy devices and gear (such as personal cold plunge tubs) and provides suggestions for sources to which you can turn for more information and to get started on your journey. Now all you have to do is read on to begin your personal cold therapy adventure.

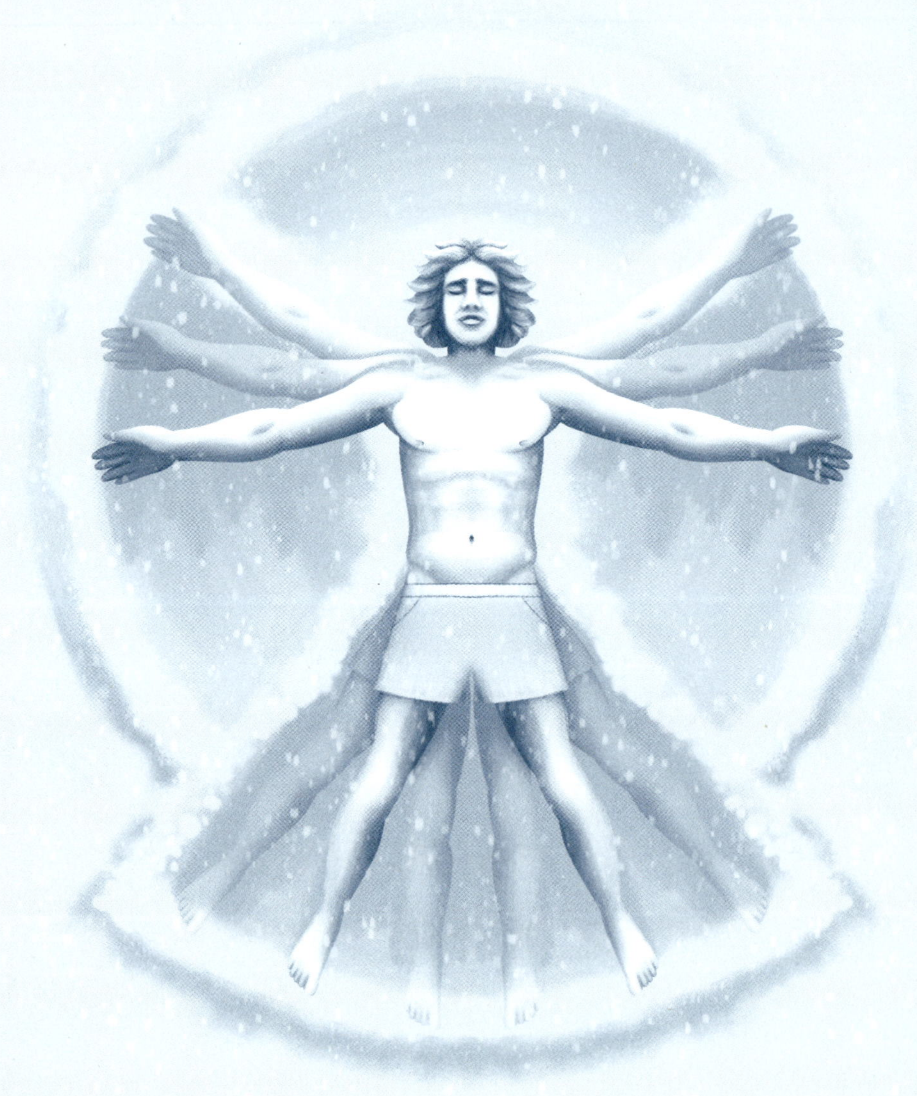

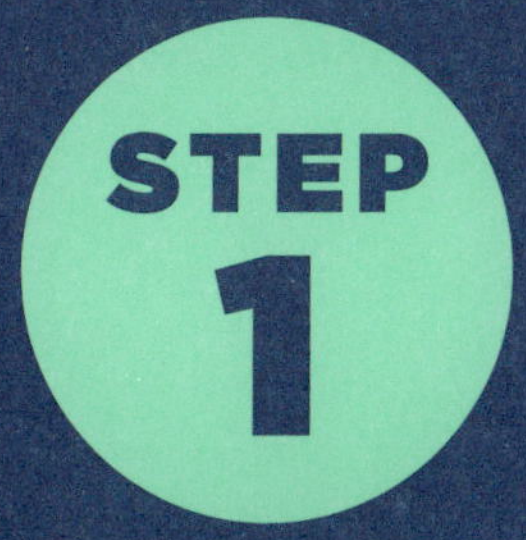

OWN THE INTEL

"Snow brings a special quality with it—the power to stop life as you know it dead in its tracks."

—NANCY HATCH WOODWARD

Cold is full of raw health potential. It can help you treat that sprained ankle or recover from knee replacement. It mutes pain signals and can even help manage certain diseases. What's more, there's a good amount of evidence that cold boosts overall wellness and makes you feel better for a significant amount of time—even after you've warmed up. All of which is why cold therapy increasingly piques the interest of both people seeking natural ways to be healthier and medical professionals and researchers who collect the real world data behind the "why." There is a lot of possible bang for the buck for something that is basically free and easy to use.

But cold therapy's easy access sometimes leads to people oversimplifying it without first doing their research. In reality, before you can just "jump in" (sometimes literally), you need to gain a basic understanding of the mechanisms at work for two main reasons: safety and efficiency. This is why an overview of the science behind cold exposure is the first step in this book.

Safety is the most important. People can and do die of extreme cold exposure. The Centers for Disease Control and Prevention (CDC) reports that 2024 saw more than 2,500 people succumb to extreme cold in the United States alone. Even more people, including experts like avid mountain climbers and wilderness survivalists, lose digits or limbs to frostbite. Cold is no joke. Our bodies just aren't built to hold up under a blast of exceptionally low temperatures without protection (or controls).

Understanding what cold does to your body will ensure you are participating safely in cold therapy without coming to any harm. The knowledge that follows will equip you to avoid detrimental effects and detect trouble signs that could indicate looming hypothermia or frostbite. If you want to keep yourself out of danger, you need to know what the red flags look like—especially because any negative side effects from cold therapy are a whole lot easier to shut down before they take hold than they are to reverse once they're in full swing.

Efficiency is the second reason to give yourself a working knowledge of the science behind cold therapy. After all, if you're going to make yourself uncomfortable, you want to get the most you can out of the therapy.

Let's be honest. Who wants to endure shivering in an ice bath or clocking time in a cold chamber without seeing some big payback? The whole point of the experience is to score major health benefits, right?

By establishing a rock-solid grasp of the fundamentals behind how cold therapy works, you can maximize your post-therapy results. The whole idea here is to make an educated choice so that you take advantage of cold therapy's true potential in both the short and long term. That knowledge will be particularly useful as you become more and more experienced and start making refinements to specifics like timing, temperature, and frequency.

Education becomes even more critical when you consider that most cold-therapy regimens are self-created and self-directed. They're just aren't a lot of medical or even sports training pros who are well-versed in the therapy or building a regimen around it. That could well be the best argument for making yourself the expert.

And remember: Bodies and reactions are different from human to human. One person's unendurable ice bath is another's rejuvenating plunge. No matter what, the science remains the same. The biology, physiology, and psychology of cold allows for a great deal of experimentation. Knowing what personal limits can be safely pushed is a matter of preference, as are which are hard guardrails will keep you safe. And insight into exactly what's happening to your body during therapy, especially at the early "shock" stage, may help you tolerate the cold for the length of time that will get you to the results you're after.

So let's dive into the science of what actually happens when your body gets cold.

YOUR BODY, CHILLED

Fortunately for anyone who slept through biology class in high school, the science behind cold's effect on the body is fairly well researched, predictable, and ruled by fundamental cause and effect. Extreme cold has an impact on just about every system, function, and tissue in your body. But it all starts on the surface because cold impacts your body from the outside in.

SKIN DEEP

Your skin is your largest organ. So, it should come as no surprise that the first reaction to low temperatures occurs in your skin. In response to cold, small blood vessels near the surface significantly narrow in a process called *vasoconstriction*. This redirects blood flow—and the heat your blood carries—from your extremities to your core. Specifically, blood flows to your torso and head. That can be a radical and disconcerting effect.

And yet, it makes sense. Your body's number-one priority is survival. Frostbite in a limb, even if it destroys a finger or a whole arm, won't immediately kill you. As long as the heart, lungs, and other internal organs continue to function, life persists. That's why, during the threat of extreme cold exposure, your body ensures blood and heat go where they're needed the most.

The cycle between cooling and warming the body revitalizes skin. As many a dermatology patient has discovered, cold therapy can be an inexpensive alternative to plastic surgery treatments like Botox and pricey skin care creams and lotions. Exposure to low temperatures spurs collagen production. That collagen has several benefits, but the most obvious is an increase in skin health. In fact, the collagen burst spurred by cold exposure has been shown to reduce skin wrinkling. Boosted blood circulation itself actually gives cold therapy adherents that much-sought-after "glow of good health."

The effect on the skin is just the start of a cascading effect that anyone who has taken a swim in cold water will recognize. Your body processes cold from the fingers and toes to the arms and legs to the head and torso, in that order. (That's why numbness in the digits is a reliable first sign that you've reached the limits of exposure and need to bring your cold therapy session to a close.)

As part of its impact on circulation, cold exposure also affects nerves on the surface of the skin. One of cold therapy's most obvious effects is to mute the signals from these nerves. That translates to a handy upside—exposure to cold actually acts as an *analgesic*, or pain reliever.

CIRCULATORY IMPACT

Blood flow doesn't just affect the skin—the "envelope"—of your body. As all those blood vessels constrict, your heart rate and blood pressure increase. This adds to the burden on your cardiovascular system; this is why it's so important that anyone with underlying heart disease or cardiopulmonary conditions consult their primary care provider or cardiologist before ever attempting cold therapy. In an otherwise healthy person, the response can actually mimic the cardio benefits of brisk exercise.

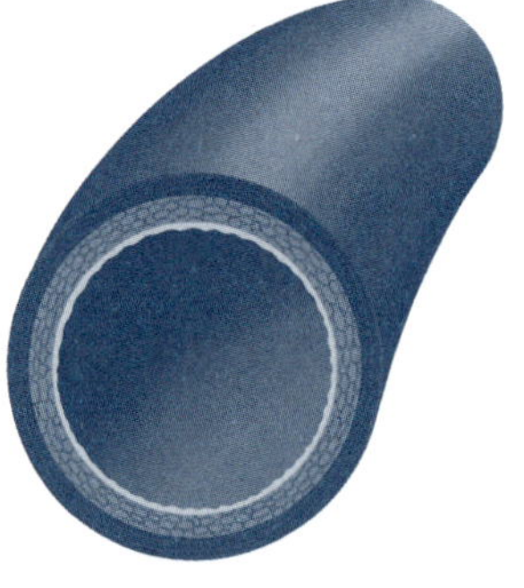

ROOM TEMPERATURE
Normal Blood Vessel

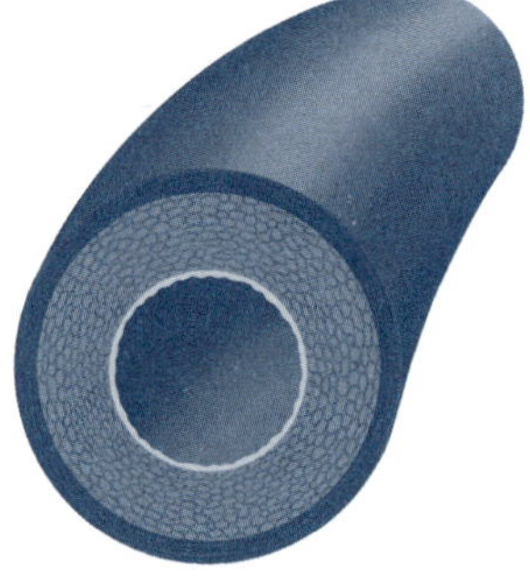

EXTREME COLD
Vasoconstriction

The Exception to the Rule: Glabrous Skin

Certain areas on your body are more sensitive than elsewhere. This is particularly true of the palms of your hands, the soles of your feet, and the upper part of your face. Those areas, and only those areas, are what's known as *glabrous tissue*. They are slightly different in structure than the skin on the rest of your body, including being hairless and containing many more sensory receptors and fine nerves than other areas of skin.

WHY DOES THAT MATTER?

Well, you feel cold more quickly on your palms and soles. More importantly, heat loss is accelerated through glabrous skin. This is why, depending on the type of cold therapy you're doing, you may want to wear special mitts or slippers or even a mask. This special gear ensures tingling or burning in your glabrous skin doesn't cause you to curtail your cold therapy before your target time.

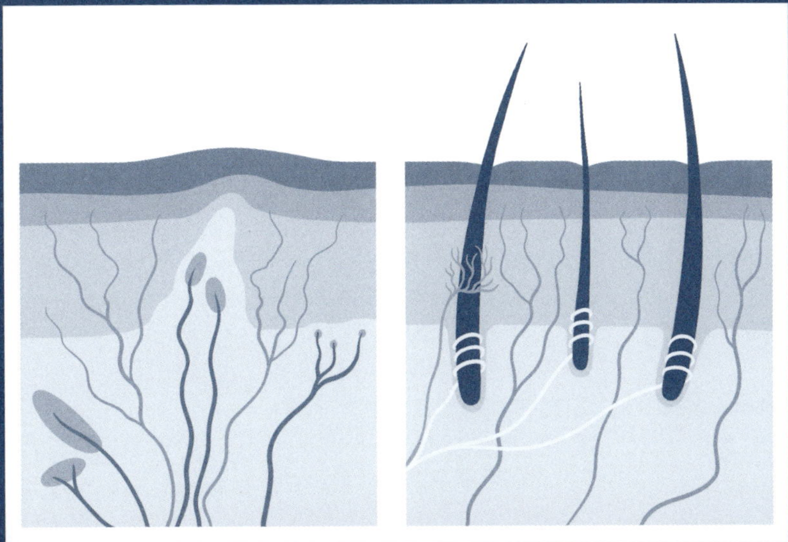

Glabrous skin (left) has far more receptors than other areas—known as "hairy skin" (right)—because glabrous skin has no hair follicles. The excess of receptors make glabrous skin conduct the feeling of cold much more quickly and sharply.

BREATHING THROUGH THE EXPERIENCE

As your blood vessels constrict in response to cold, your breathing becomes shallow and rapid. This is what's known as the "cold shock response" (if you've ever gasped out loud after jumping into an unexpectedly chilly swimming pool, you'll completely understand that description). The initial response is your reaction to the jolt to your system, and it can actually lead to hyperventilation if you do not take steps to control your breathing. Regardless, breathing will continue to be labored because the cold air in the surrounding environment narrows your airways and irritates the throat and lung linings.

Spending time in any cold therapy that involves whole-body exposure will involve moderating your breathing to one degree or another. A plunge in an ice bath or a swim in an icy lake won't last long if you can't slow and control your breath, bringing it back to some semblance of normal. That explains why cold therapy is often coupled with breathwork—exercises that help you consciously control your breathing.

Conscious breathwork is an important part of the Wim Hof Method, the cold therapy named for the extreme-cold advocate and health influencer. Wim Hof uses controlled breathing to moderate the impact of cold immersion, and he exploits it to optimize the beneficial effects of his particular brand of cold therapy (which is not for everyone and certainly not for the faint of heart).

The crucial takeaway is, no matter what type of whole-body cold therapy you might try, how you breathe will largely determine how well you handle the experience and the duration of your exposure.

NERVOUS SYSTEM STRESS RESPONSE

Breathing is just one part of a much more complex nervous system reaction to the sudden systemic stress of whole-body exposure to extreme cold. That word "stress" is key.

Exposure to cold is a stress on your body and mind, and initiates many of the reactions that other stressors cause. We tend to think of all stress as "bad" (job deadlines, financial worries) and unhealthy. But there are

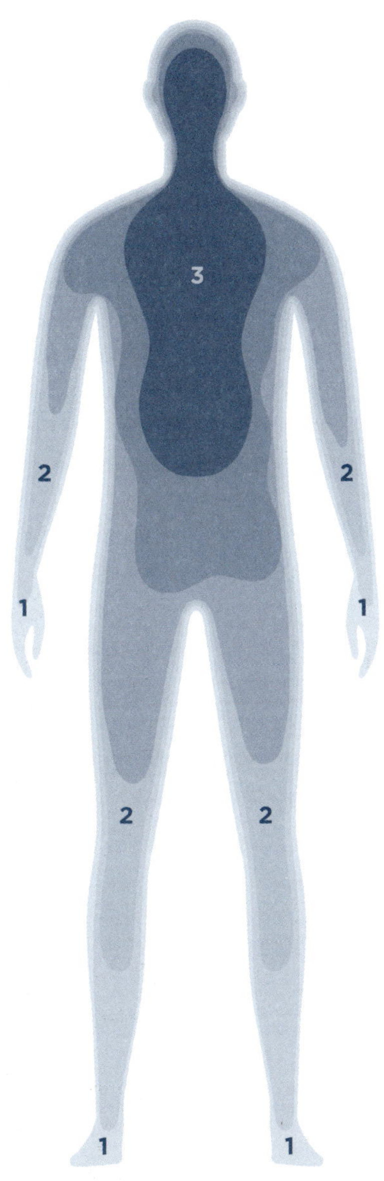

Order of body-chilling when exposed to cold

many types of stress (like the excitement of starting a new job or pushing the limits of a workout to get past a plateau) and some can be beneficial. Control stress, and you can use it to grow and improve.

The body and brain's stress response to cold is unusually complex and can seem contradictory because the response involves both the parasympathetic and the sympathetic systems—opposite sides that make up the autonomic nervous system. That system as a whole controls all those functions we take for granted but don't consciously have to initiate or control, for instance, breathing and sweating. The parasympathetic acts in opposition to the sympathetic system, creating a soothing and restorative state called the "rest-and-digest" response. The opposing sympathetic system is famous for the "fight-or-flight" reaction that sends all our bodily systems into overdrive.

The nervous system's initial reaction to immersing yourself in icy water or exposing your whole body to the hyper-chilled air in the cryochamber is to fire up the sympathetic system. That floods your bloodstream with stress hormones—most notably, adrenaline and noradrenaline (also called *epinephrine* and *norepinephrine*). Breathing quickens, pulse rate jumps, and all the reactions you would expect when faced with danger happen in quick succession.

But those reactions are mediated by the concurrent stimulation of your vagus nerve. Cold powerfully affects nerves throughout the body, including the vagus. This large and important nerve starts in the medulla oblongata region in your brain and travels down through your torso to your gut. Essentially, it serves as the body's internal messaging application, acting as the conduit for vital communications from the gastrointestinal tract, circulatory system, and internal organs up to the brain. By transmitting these key signals, the nerve plays an important role in regulating crucial functions ranging from digestion to hormone levels to heart rate and even mood. It is largely responsible for activating the parasympathetic system.

The stimulation of the vague nerve allows you to balance your initial sympathetic system reaction (fight or flight) to the shock of cold with a more relaxed and calm state. At least you can, if you manage to stick with

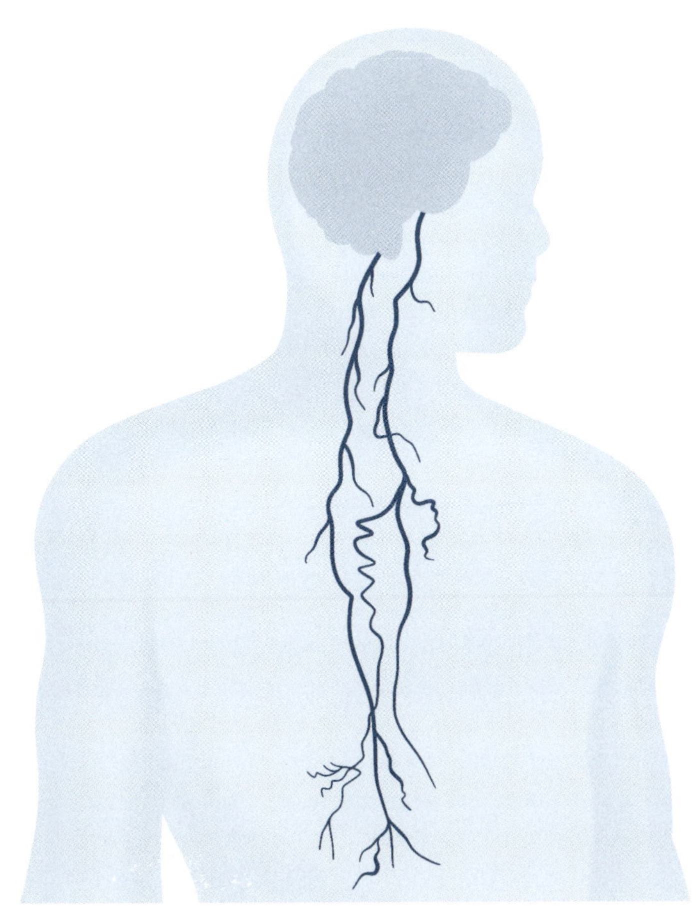

The path of the vagus nerve

the cold therapy and not get out (which is exactly what the sympathetic system is screaming at you to do!).

Hyped-Up Hormones

There's a lot going on in your nervous system during whole-body cold therapy. The hormones produced are perhaps the most powerful part of those responses.

Your brain and glands react to extreme low temperatures by releasing adrenaline, noradrenaline, and dopamine, among many other "neuromodulators." The first two are traditional stress hormones that amp up energy and awareness. Dopamine is the feel-good hormone. It mediates the effects of the other two to some degree. That's why cold therapy can simultaneously wake you up and make you feel calmer. You become more alert, and your mood improves, so you relax at the same time as your mental focus heightens.

It's important to note that, in practice, the effects of those hormones last for a significant period of time, even after you're finished with your cold therapy. Someone who does whole-body cold immersion in the morning will still feel energized and experience a sense of well-being several hours later. That's why experts advise against doing cold therapy in the evening. The "wide-awake" mental state is one of the most obvious effects of cold therapy. Thanks to those stress hormones, cold exposure can be a better "wake-me-up" than a double espresso!

The jolt of cold immersion literally amps up the brain's processing and directs your adrenal glands to release the hormones that make you feel focused and energized. This may seem like a modest benefit, but it influences everything from how productive you are at work to how safe a driver you are. A small British study found that a five-minute cold-water immersion created a measurable increase in alertness and mental focus. Maybe just as importantly, the test subjects reported a perceptible decrease in anxiety.

However, the mental alertness spurred by cold therapy follows a bell curve. Expose yourself to extreme cold for too long and not only does the effect wane but your condition will start to trend in the opposite direction.

Eventually, you will begin to experience the first stages of hypothermia, which include mental confusion, trouble thinking rationally, and even panic.

Cold therapy doesn't just affect adrenaline and noradrenaline; controlled cold exposure has a significant impact on a range of hormones. A number of those come into play as the body attempts to burn calories and heat itself. For instance, there is evidence to suggest that regular cold therapy may spur hormones that have a positive effect on blood glucose levels, lipids, and amino acids.

Cold exposure also spurs the release of endorphins, essentially the body's version of opioids. This accounts for the euphoria that many regular cold swimmers and whole-body cold therapy advocates report feeling during and for some time after sessions. Endorphins also amplify the pain-killing properties of cold therapy.

Stress Response as a Tool

All of these reactions and processes that happen in the nervous system during cold exposure are part of our bodies' stress response, and intentionally activating them can actually be a good thing. Many of us think of stress as a purely mental state. But stress is much more complicated than that. And while excessive stress caused by negative stressors can be detrimental to your health (both mental and physical), stress can also be a highly useful tool in improving your fitness, performance, and well-being in a number of ways.

Hormesis is the adaptive response to stress. Think of it this way: You stress your muscles when you do an hour on a severe incline treadmill. They need to recuperate, but the result of repeatedly stressing them in this fashion is that they adapt to the workload, and you improve your time and distance and can tackle bigger challenges. The muscles have adapted.

This adaptive progression is part of a cold therapy regimen as well. The idea is to stress your cells by exposing your body to cold (but not so much that you do damage). One 2024 study found that, in as few as four cold-water plunges, subjects had a reduction in cellular stress and boosted the cellular defensive mechanism called *autophagy*. That process is incredibly powerful in the body, repairing damaged proteins and other cellular structures. This means exposure in a controlled and ongoing fashion can translate to the body working harder to heal itself and protect you even more against disease.

The stress response also improves your general physical tolerance to low temperatures and helps you adapt to endure even colder temperatures for longer times.

This effect, though, isn't just related to cold. Because there is such a significant mental and psychological impact from cold exposure, hormesis works its magic on your psychological state as well. This is a key, poorly understood but potentially incredibly valuable side benefit of cold therapy: You can become more mentally and emotionally resilient in the face of challenges.

THE BODY AS ITS OWN FURNACE

When you get really cold, your body works hard trying to warm itself back up. The most important area the body protects is your core temperature. The complicated process by which your body maintains your core temperature is called *thermoregulation*, and it can be exploited to serve your goals in several different ways.

Let's start with how the body perceives temperature fluctuations. Your internal "thermostat" is located in the brain. The hypothalamus region is responsible for *homeostasis*, or keeping your body's systems in balance with each other and the environment around you. That includes adjusting your core temperature to keep the body and its organs operating as they should. This is why most cold therapies avoid directly cooling the head. Chill that part of your brain, and the thermostat can be fooled into firing up your furnace and, ironically, may cause overheating and dehydration.

As your body chills, thermoregulation escalates, and the body fights diligently to keep that core temperature up. That effort consumes a lot of calories, which is why weight loss can be a component of a regular cold therapy regimen. There also are related effects, such as converting white fat to beige or brown fat, which will be discussed further in Step 2 (see page 70).

Suffice it to say that keeping the body working to maintain core temperature provides several health benefits and is why reheating after cold therapy should be done slowly and from the inside out. You want the body to keep working to heat itself, burning even more calories in the process. Thermoregulation, however, is not the only way for the body to heat itself.

Moving Muscles

As many a pro athlete can testify, cold therapy holds the potential to help muscles recover from athletic exertion. But even if you're not an athlete, your muscles will be affected by cold therapy exposure.

Involuntary shivering is, in fact, the first and most obvious sign that cold is taking its toll on your body. This muscle action is the body's attempt at generating its own heat. By simply being active, you, too, can generate your own heat. It's why cold therapy advocates who use cold pools or natural bodies of water as their medium of choice start vigorously swimming as soon as they get in. In those cases, exercise substitutes for the involuntary shivering (and usually feels better).

This use of muscles—voluntary or not—increases the calorie-burning potential of any cold therapy. That's one of the reasons many people, including research professionals, believe that cold therapy can be effective for weight loss. However, before you charge into a marathon ice-bath session to try to drop a few pounds, it's wise to keep in mind that *uncontrollable* shivering is also an early warning sign of hypothermia.

The muscles in your limbs are the first to be affected by extremes of cold and are where you'll notice the impact the most. Your muscles will be starved of blood supply; nerve signals will be blocked; and muscle tissue will become, literally, stiff and unresponsive. As you're exposed to low temperatures over time, you'll start to feel weaker than normal. Your reaction time will slow. You'll move sluggishly and become clumsier. Those are all clear indicators that it's time to end your cold therapy session.

COMPLEX INTERACTIONS

Although the body and brain's responses to cold exposure are well-documented and fairly well understood physiological processes, there's a good deal that even seasoned medical researchers and avid enthusiasts don't know about the intertwined physical effects of this health practice.

It can be difficult to study cold therapy subjects over long time periods. However, there are many logical and reasonable conclusions we can draw from available scientific knowledge and real-world experience. Some intertwined effects on the body include:

Boosted immune system: Sudden immersion in extremely cold water stimulates special infection-fighting blood cells called *leukocytes*. It also spurs an increase in other infection-fighting cells, such as *monocytes*. Potentially even more exciting, one 1999 study found that cold exposure boosted the number of circulating natural killer cells. One purpose of these specialized white blood cells is to hunt down and destroy cancer cells. Cold therapy could potentially contribute to cancer prevention and even work alongside cancer treatments such as chemotherapy and radiation to bolster results.

Aging (or not): Intact bodies have been found above 8,000 feet (2.4 km) of elevation on Mount Everest decades after the climbers got lost or stranded in storms and succumbed to hypothermia. Their bodies were nearly perfectly preserved. That illustrates the intriguing possibility that less severe cold applied more strategically and for a limited time period might slow the cellular process of aging. On a more superficial level, cold stimulates collagen production. Since your body produces less collagen as you age, any boost to collagen levels will keep skin smooth and elastic, creating a more youthful appearance.

Active mitochondria: Experts and researchers are also looking into cold therapy's role in activating mitochondria. Mitochondria are complicated organelles aptly called the "powerhouses of cells." That's because they produce the energy cells throughout the body needed to function properly. By stimulating mitochondria proliferation, cold therapy may make energy production more efficient and boost cellular health over the long term. However, this is theoretical. That idea has yet to be fully studied.

THE LOGISTICS OF COLD

Now that you know the effects of cold therapy on your body, it's time to dive in—pun intended—to the logistical details you need to know before doing cold therapy. We'll start with the most important variables you'll deal with in establishing your own cold therapy regimen. These are, in order of importance, the temperature, time spent exposed (either in water or in air), and the frequency and schedule of the regimen.

THERMOMETER, CLOCK, AND CALENDAR

Temperature is sometimes referred to as "intensity" in cold therapy studies and among advocates. Depending on the setting and type of cold therapy you use, you may not have much control over the actual temperature. So it is important to always measure the temperature of whatever medium you use—whether it's an icy lake, a cryochamber, or a gym-based ice bath—so you can correctly adjust the time you spend in the therapy and chart your progress. Although your body fat (a natural insulator) and other factors like age, gender, and fitness will impact your cold temperature of choice, the generally accepted ideal range for most cold therapy is 50°F to 60°F (10°C to 15°C) in the water, or -85°F to -140°F (-65°C to -96°C) in the air.

When it comes to cold exposure, temperature is always partnered with time. It is essential to track the amount of time you have been exposed to the cold. Overexposure can quickly spiral into a dangerous situation, and warming your body back to a safe and stable temperature is not as simple as just removing yourself from the water or cold environment. Always measure the amount of time you're spending in whatever type of cold therapy you choose. You'll find specific time recommendations for different practices, in Step 4.

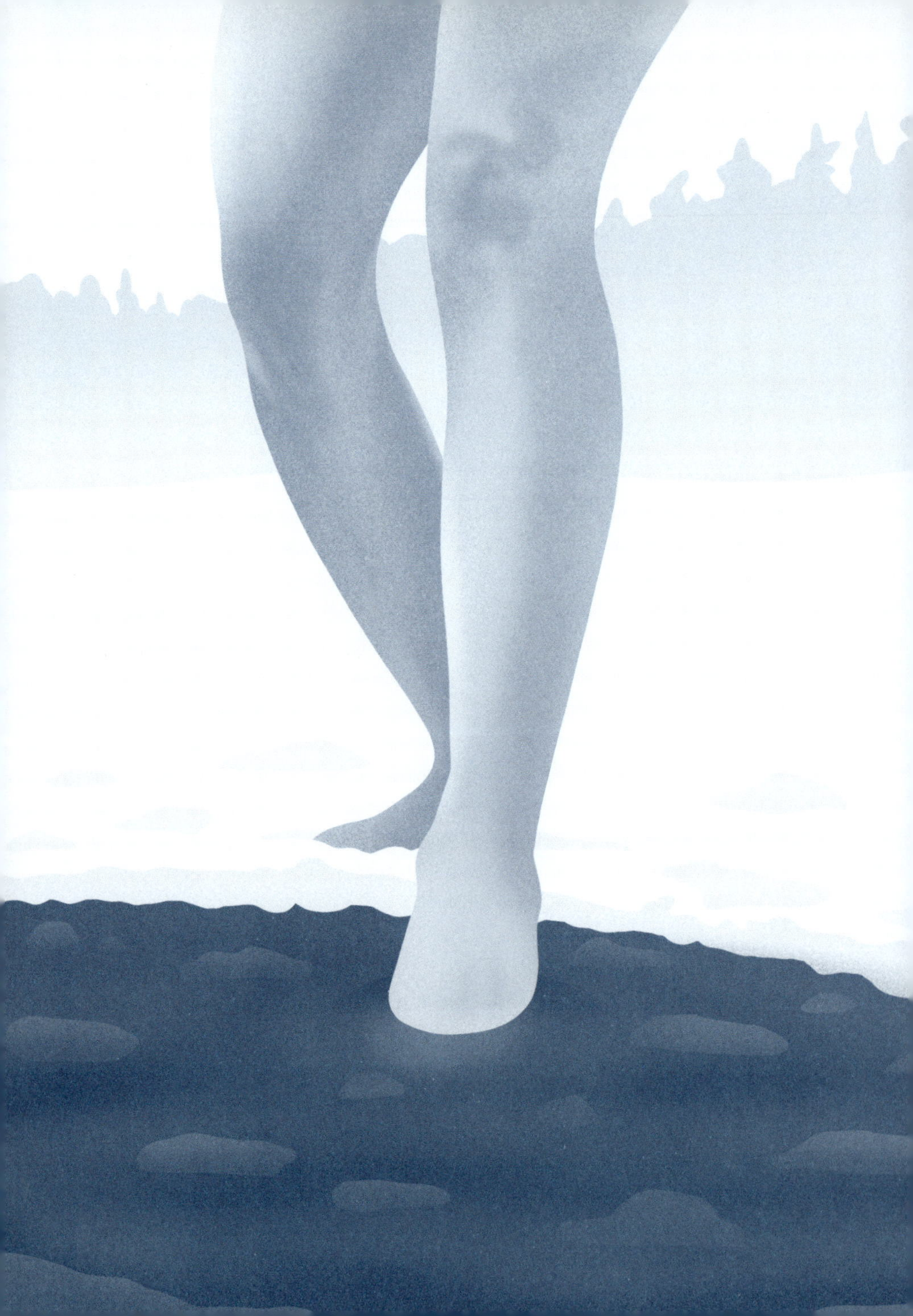

Frequency is the third logistic to consider before jumping into your cold therapy—and it is the most imprecise factor. Although cold therapy advocates recommend sessions two to three times per week as an average, this recommendation varies widely. High-performance athletes who work out five or more days a week, for instance, will often take ice baths after every workout in their pre-season. (They normally reduce the number drastically during the competitive season.) The frequency you ultimately choose for your cold therapy regimen will depend on your schedule and the type of cold therapy you choose and how accessible it is. Over time, you may make adjustments to the frequency of your sessions to better achieve your goals. However, shoot for at least two times per week to have a measurable impact on your body that will allow you to gather data you can track, analyze, and use to refine your practice.

GENDER AND AGE

There is a strong personal element in establishing any cold therapy regimen. Your preferences and comfort will no doubt play a role the type of cold therapy you choose, and the realities of your day-to-day life will guide the specifics of time, temperature, and scheduling.

But two other crucial variables to consider are gender and age.

On average, men have greater muscle mass than women do. That means they produce more internal heat. It is no surprise then, that women will feel extreme low temperatures more sharply. A 2018 study backs this up. Researchers found that women begin to shiver at temperatures four degrees warmer than those at which men do. The takeaway is that you may need to adjust your cold therapy from the recommendations in this book or of any professional you're consulting.

Age also plays a role in how cold affects you. As we grow older, we tend to lose some types of body fat. This means our bodies are less insulated, and cold will likely impact us more than when we were younger. You've likely seen this effect in action if you've spent time with elderly relatives; they inevitably need the thermostat set higher than younger people do. They are literally more sensitive to cold.

COLD WATER VERSUS COLD AIR THERAPIES

So now that you know the variables associated with cold therapy, let's explore the methodologies available to you for putting that knowledge into practice. When most people think of cold therapy, they automatically picture dunking into water or ice. But as the practice has grown in popularity, so have the options. Now, cold-air immersion is also a possibility. As you can imagine, water and air create extremely different cold therapy experiences.

Cold water conducts heat away from your body much quicker and more efficiently than cold air does. In fact, you lose body heat almost four times faster when immersed in cold water, as opposed to being exposed to air that is chilled to that same temperature. This is important if you've already become accustomed to cold water therapy and are considering using a cold-air cryochamber; the cold air will need to be a significantly lower temperature than the water to achieve the same effect.

A regulated cold-air environment—such as a cryochamber—gives you much finer control over your cold therapy experience than, say, a plunge in an ice bath would. As a result, exposure to cold water can lead to hypothermia much quicker whereas cold-air immersion units can be adjusted to within a degree or two of a target temperature.

Of course, cold-air therapies vary depending on the option you choose. The crudest version is simply to spend time outdoors underdressed on a cold day. That's not particularly precise or controllable, and results will certainly vary. The more cutting-edge alternative is a cryochamber. These are slowly growing in popularity for their convenience and because some people find cold-air exposure preferable to the jarring experience of an icy plunge. The largest chambers resemble a small sauna that you step inside and either stand or sit in while cold air is circulated around you. Some models are small cylinders and enclose the body in a standing or sitting position, so that the head is out of the cold. Others are cabinets that enclose around you as you sit and seal around your neck so that your head is outside of the unit. (Units that allow the head to protrude are called *cryosaunas* in the industry.) Most of these are too expensive to consider for home use, but a growing number of clinics and upscale gyms offer them.

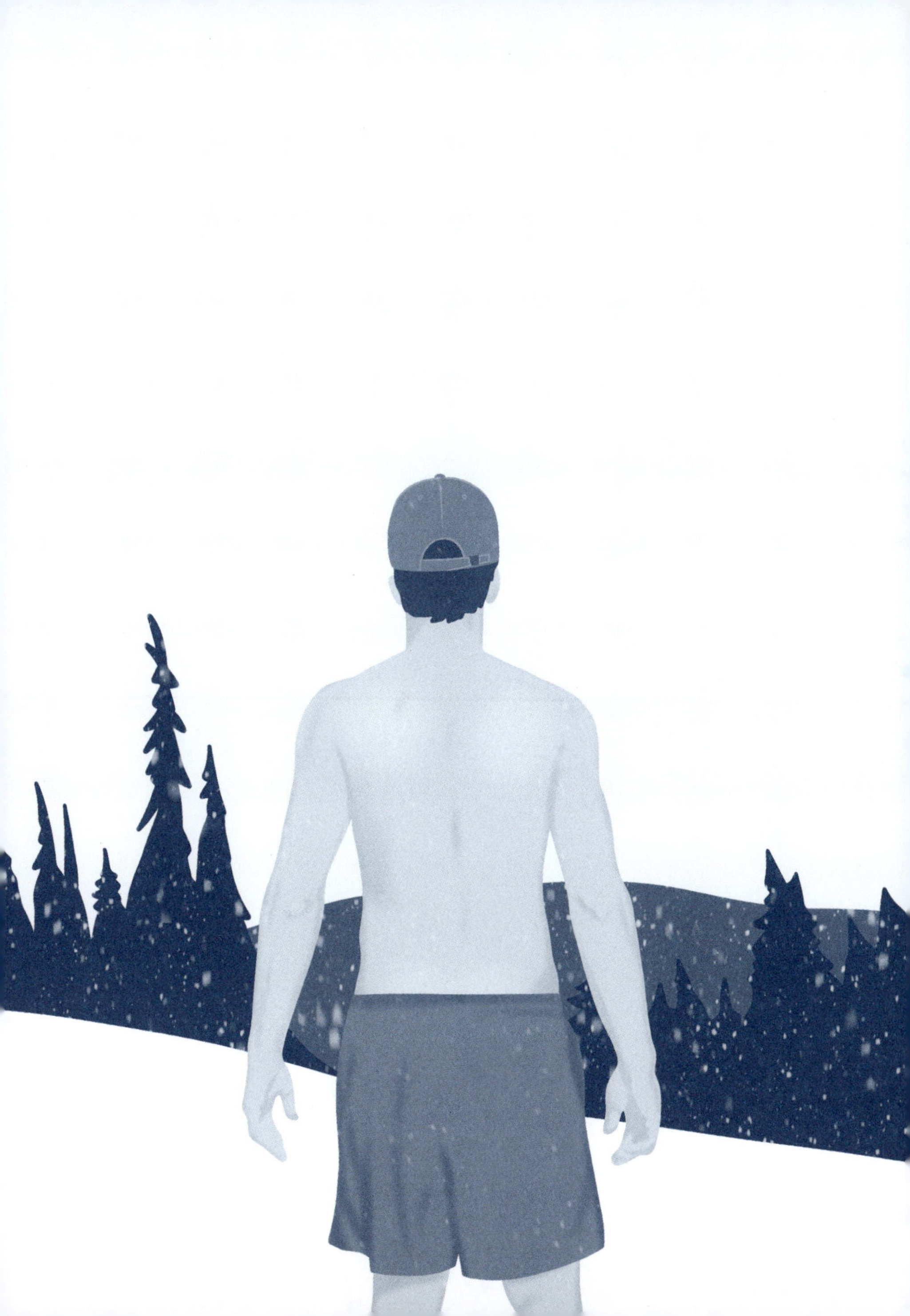

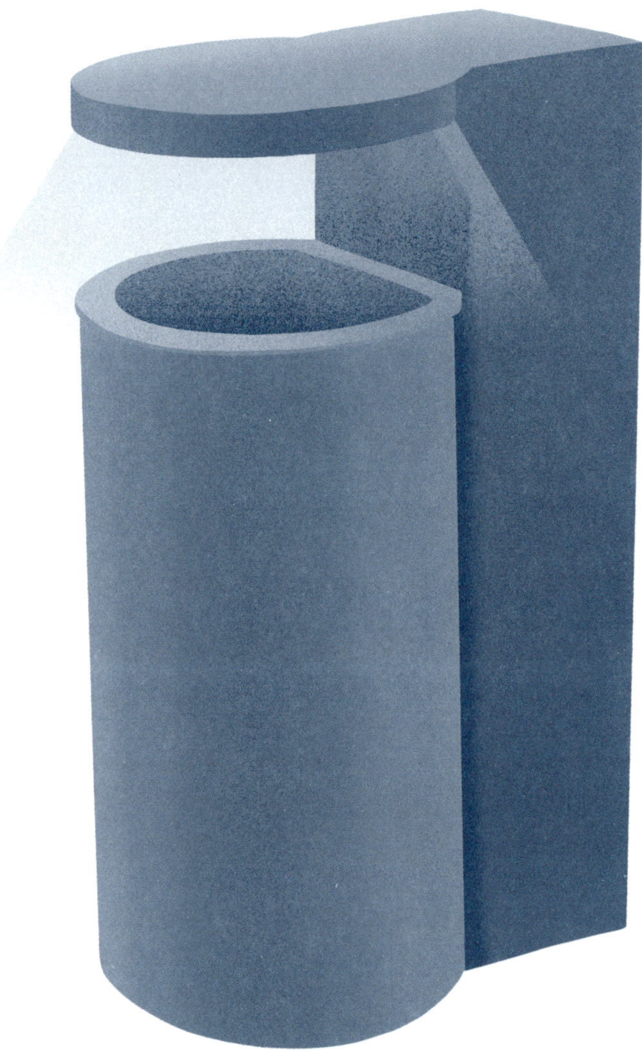

Cryosaunas typically allow the head to protrude while cold air is circulated around the body. These are becoming more common in high-end gyms and other wellness facilities.

Choosing between air and water exposure is a matter of personal preference, comfort, and availability. But as more and more studies compare the impact of cold air to that of cold water, your decision may be guided by what cold therapy is best for the results you're after. For instance, a 2016 study found that post-exercise cold-water immersion was measurably more effective in boosting recovery among competitive bicyclists than cold-air exposure was. The caveat here, as elsewhere in the book, is that a great deal of research still needs to be done comparing the two and their respective effects on specific conditions, diseases, trauma, and athletic or injury recovery.

SMALL PART VERSUS WHOLE-BODY EXPOSURE

The physiological changes that happen during cold therapy described earlier in Step 1 reflect cold exposure over all or most of the body. But there are many types of cold therapy that focus on a more modest surface area. Applications like post-surgery cold-water cuffs, specialized wearables for knee conditions, and cryotherapy devices used to treat acne or other dermatological conditions are more self-contained and controllable. Simply put, whole-body exposure (up to the neck) is a more powerful cold therapy than cold showers or targeted versions like knee cuffs.

The effects of focal point treatments are localized and simpler. That makes them easier to measure against target goals. They either improve the condition you're treating or they don't, so the results are easy to judge. Focal point cold therapy is usually done under the guidance of a medical expert, so specifics like timing and frequency have been worked out. Sophisticated modern focal point treatment devices and options are precise and well-engineered, which limits the potential for any tissue damage. Unlike the trial-and-error needed to determine your personal ideal time in an ice bath or cold shower, focal treatments are often prescribed with exact directions for use.

Focal point options don't offer the potentially system-wide benefits that whole-body exposure might. The main concern with any local treatment is frostbite. That's why, whether you're using a post-surgery cuff or an ice pack, you should never expose the skin directly to the source of cold. In all cases, you also carefully moderate both temperature and time (in concert with one another).

LONG-TERM EFFECTS OF COLD THERAPY

Many people who "take the plunge" into cold therapy become enthusiasts who establish regular exposure routines. Some even consider it a lifelong practice. Obviously, how much you embrace—or don't—your own cold therapy experience will depend on the type of cold therapy you choose and how successful it is in delivering the results you're after.

Some types are meant to be temporary. For example, a cold-water cuff for surgery recovery is a short-term treatment. Other cold-therapy regimens beg to be made part of a routine. Swimming in a cold lake or the ocean as part of a club can easily become a regular and happy ritual. It can be as much a social occasion as a health treatment. Given the role of social interaction in maintaining wellness, that can be considered a core benefit as well.

Even though we don't know with certainty the long-term health benefits in relation to the amount of time spent engaging in a cold therapy regimen, we do know that the physical and psychological impact lingers for hours. Abundant anecdotal evidence suggests the upsides persist even longer than that. These include:

Mental well-being: Getting in the habit of a regular cold therapy regimen may have significant mental health benefits. Perhaps the most apparent is day-to-day improvement of mood, alertness, and mental focus. Enthusiasts suggest you'll feel better in the long-term. That's a difficult thing to measure, much less study, but there is abundant anecdotal evidence to support the idea.

Slimming down: Obtaining a healthier body mass index (BMI) may be a significant result of regular cold therapy. Cold exposure triggers noradrenaline that floods white fat cells, in turn converting them into adipose tissue

A Brief History of Cold Therapy

The idea of using cold for health and healing is far from new. It dates back to ancient Egypt, where evidence shows that practitioners used cold compresses to reduce the trauma of infection and wounds.

300 BCE

The father of modern medicine himself, the Greek physician Hippocrates, used snow or ice to reduce inflammation and treat skin diseases. He documented the potential that cold exposure had to reduce swelling, slow bleeding, and lessen pain. Ancient Roman baths even offered cold plunges to relieve pain and improve circulation.

1812

Cold therapy was further explored through the lens of war and the gruesome injuries resulting from battle. Napoleon's chief surgeon packed ice around critically wounded limbs before amputating them—reducing pain and potentially fatal blood loss. The practice was widely adopted from that point on.

1819

Sometimes called the "Father of Cryosurgery," British physician James Arnett used extreme cold—a result of mixing salt and crushed ice—to freeze and destroy diseased tissue. Arnett treated many conditions with this method, including certain cancerous tumors. He later championed cold to treat skin diseases and headaches.

1950s

Post-World War II, liquid nitrogen became widely available and was used by doctors to treat various skin conditions.

1961

The development of the "ice scalpel" by British physician Irving Cooper accelerated modern wart removal and other forms of cryosurgery. Essentially a tube delivering liquid nitrogen to targeted areas, the ice scalpel was used to treat neurological disease by killing brain and tumor tissue. Cooper's work led to the term "cryosurgery."

1978

Dr. Toshima Yamaguchi built on earlier developments by expanding the use of cold exposure to treat the entire body. He effectively used his "whole-body cryotherapy" to treat pain, specifically from arthritis.

2011

Wim Hof introduced the Wim Hof Method, an extreme form of cold therapy coupled with breathwork and meditation, on the back of a Dutch study that researched the method and its potential benefits. The extreme-cold advocate went on to write several books describing his approach to cold therapy.

(beige or brown fat, in lay terms). This tissue has multiple advantages over white fat and can contribute to higher energy levels and weight loss. (You'll find a more in-depth explanation of this process under "Goal: Support or Promote Weight Loss" on page 70.)

Immunity boosting: Cold therapy has been shown to foster the production of several types of immune system cells. Primarily, these include leukocytes, monocytes, and natural killer cells. That means that regular cold therapy may help fight everything from bacterial infections to colds and even more serious viruses.

Blood sugar: Over time, cold therapy can increase insulin sensitivity. Insulin sensitivity is key to preventing the onset of type 2 diabetes and heading off other blood sugar issues.

Now, despite all of these health benefits, cold therapy is not without its risks. That's why you should always proceed with caution when engaging in the practice, whether you're partaking in one session or scheduling a full regimen. Before we wrap up this chapter, let's look at some of the risk associated with overexposing your body to cold.

THE TOLL OF OVEREXPOSURE

To fully understand cold therapy, it's essential to understand the specific dangers that anyone doing cold therapy may encounter. Cold numbs. That's both a good and a bad thing. It's the reason that cold therapy can provide pain relief. But it also means that the practice can mask damage from overexposure without you realizing you're spending too long immersed or exposed. This is why it's important to ease into any cold therapy regimen, so that you gain an understanding of your personal limits (you'll find more specifics on how to do that in Step 4, see page 105). So, let's look at some of the risks posed by too much cold exposure:

Hypothermia: In the simplest terms, hypothermia is a condition in which the body loses heat faster than it can produce it. Technically, it occurs when your core temperature falls below 95°F (35°C). Make no mistake—this is a dangerous and potentially deadly condition. In the extreme cases it can lead to organ failure and death. The paradox of cold therapy is that the initial phase can mimic hypothermia. Ironically, symptoms of hypothermia also increase the difficulty of detecting the condition. They include uncontrollable involuntary shivering, which also happens to be a result of starting almost any cold therapy. The more worrisome red flags are neurological. Those involve difficulty thinking clearly, slurred speech, and a lack of coordination. As the condition advances, breathing slows, and you become very sleepy. Any symptom of hypothermia is a sign to stop the therapy and modify it going forward. This is the primary reason why it's so crucial to follow the safety guidelines on page 101.

Frostbite: This is perhaps the most obvious sign that you've spent too much time in the cold. Toes and fingers are the body parts most susceptible to frostbite. Early indications include cold, hard, waxy skin; pain as the area warms up; and especially a tingling "pins-and-needles" or burning sensation. There may also be a persistent redness. Soak the affected digits in lukewarm water or warm them with a heating pad set to medium low. Any sign of frostbite is an indication to stop cold therapy entirely until the area is healed. Consult your primary care provider before continuing with the therapy and modify the therapy to reduce your exposure time and intensity.

Skin and nerve damage: In rare cases, overexposure during cold therapy can result in persistent symptoms after the therapy has ended. Damaged skin may be red or white and remain numb or tingle long after you have warmed up. If that occurs, stop your cold therapy regimen and consult your primary care provider.

Although some discomfort and reddening in fingers and toes is a part of most cold therapy regimens, the signs of potential frostbite are more pronounced and linger after you've ended the therapy.

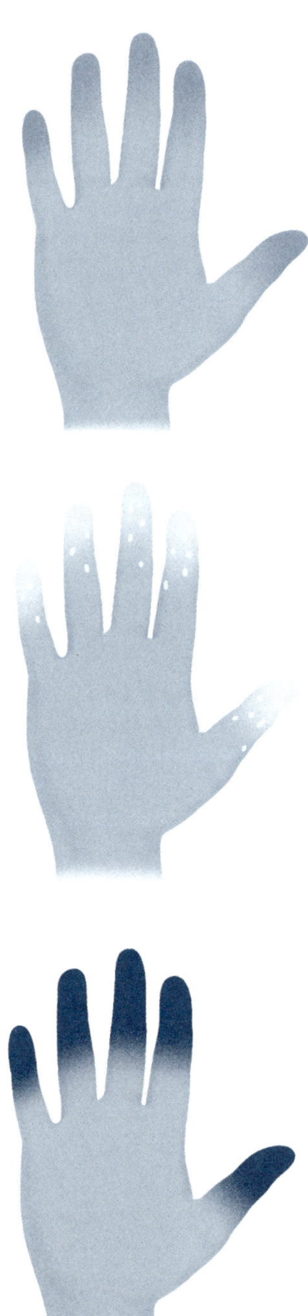

Know the Danger: Four Stages of Cold Water Immersion (CWI)

First responders and researchers have defined four distinct stages the human body goes through when immersed in water below 60°F (15°C). They offer a physiology road map to anyone engaging in whole-body water-based cold therapy. It's especially important to be aware of these signs if you are engaging in cold swims in lakes, rivers, or the ocean.

1. **Cold shock (immediately after immersion to five minutes):** This is your initial physiological response to submerging your body in water that is colder than 60°F (15°C). This stage is marked most noticeably by that initial "gasp" that is a universal reaction to cold immersion. Your breathing becomes rapid and can lead to hyperventilation unless you take steps to generate body heat (usually through activity) and control your breathing—something you can do with the breathwork described on page 106. Your blood vessels constrict and heart rate increases.

2. **Swim failure (five to thirty minutes after immersion):** Reflexes and manual dexterity begin to falter. Swimming will become noticeably harder. You're clumsier and less coordinated, which is obviously a concern if you're in deep water or are alone. Your breathing becomes more rapid and shallower than normal—unless you make a conscious effort to control it.

3. **Hypothermia (after about thirty minutes, although it may occur earlier):** This is the critical phase in which, simply put, your body loses heat faster than it can produce it. Your internal organs are cooling to dangerously low temperatures. How quickly this phase progresses depends on what you're wearing and how active you are in the water. In any case, it's a sign to get out.

4. **Collapse (any time after hypothermia onset):** This is often called the "post-rescue" phase because the symptoms are common to victims pulled out of the water by first responders. Your body struggles to survive the cold exposure. This phase includes traumatic and scary indications. Blood pressure drops abnormally low, and your muscles may not work. You may be in and out of consciousness. Unless you're warmed up rapidly and correctly, cardiac arrest or organ failure are distinct possibilities.

CONTRAINDICATIONS

While in general the health benefits of cold therapy make it worth pursuing, there are some preexisting conditions that may preclude engaging in cold therapy. They include:

Cold urticaria: This reaction to cold exposure mimics an allergic response. It can range from a mild and brief skin rash, to whole-body hives, welts, and swelling. If you notice a skin reaction to your first cold therapy session, consult a dermatologist. Generally, anyone suffering from cold urticaria will have a difficult time following a regular regimen of cold therapy, although antihistamines can moderate the response.

Raynaud's syndrome: Raynaud's causes a reduction in blood flow to the arms and legs and particularly affects the fingers and toes. Although not caused by cold, if undiagnosed this condition can mimic some of the symptoms of frostbite. Raynaud's syndrome symptoms include extreme sensitivity to cold or stress. When aggravated, Raynaud's will cause fingers and toes to turn from white to red, with accompanying numbness or tingling. If you have Raynaud's, you may already suspect that you're hypersensitive to cold. Regardless, anytime you have a severe reaction to a cold therapy session, stop the therapy, and consult your primary care provider.

BUILDING ON THE SCIENCE

The science behind cold therapy may, at first blush, seem complex. Really, though, it boils down to understanding how your body is reacting, so that you can keep yourself safe and accurately judge results. Understanding the science gives you a leg up in optimizing any cold therapy you do. But it's just as important to tune into your body, because the impact isn't just physical and data driven; it's mental, relative, and qualitative.

Now that you know the science behind cold therapy, the next step is for you to identify your own health goals, which will determine the best cold therapy method going forward. In the next step, we'll zero in on these goals to ensure the type of cold therapy you pick for your regimen achieves the results you're after.

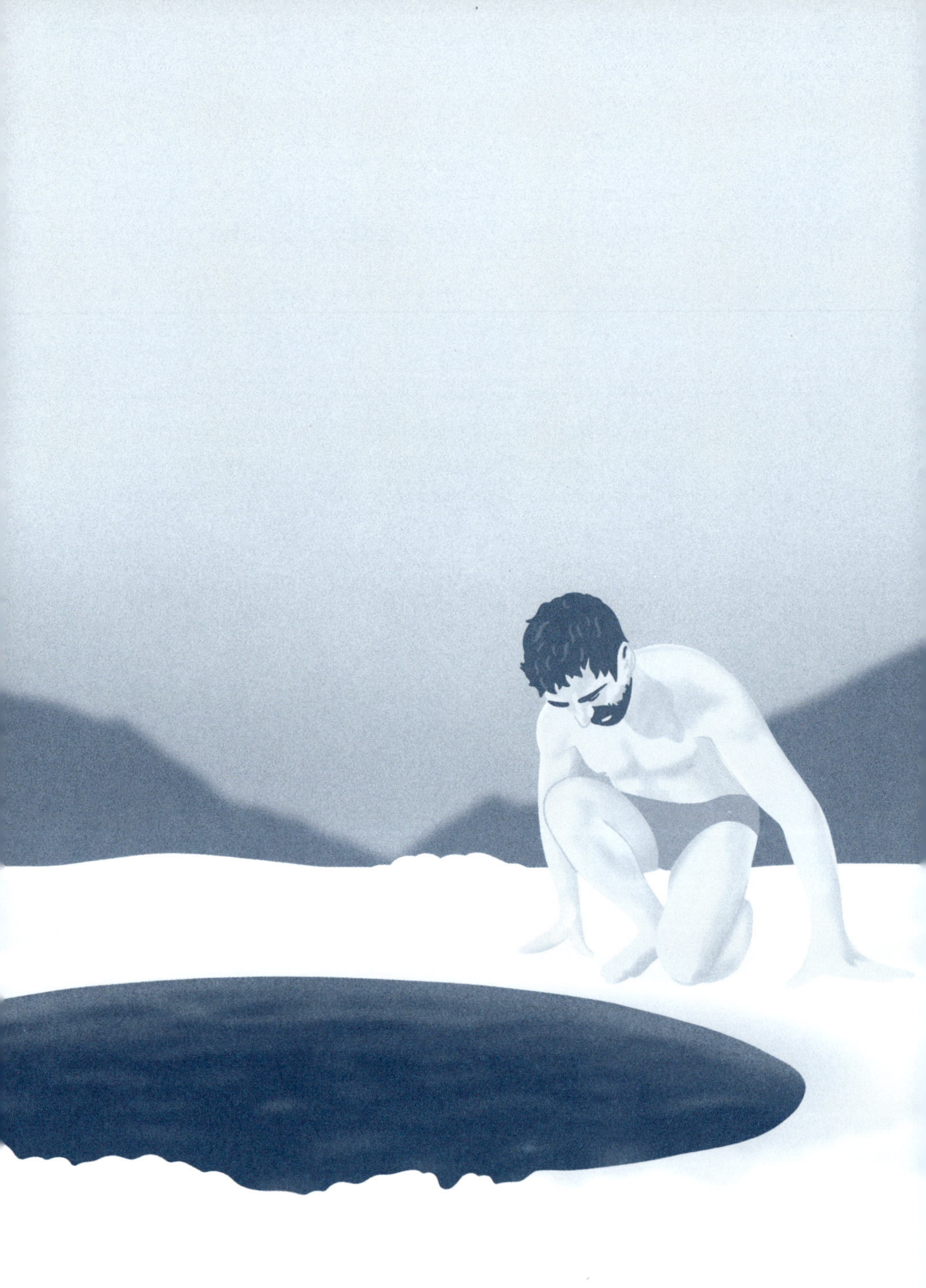

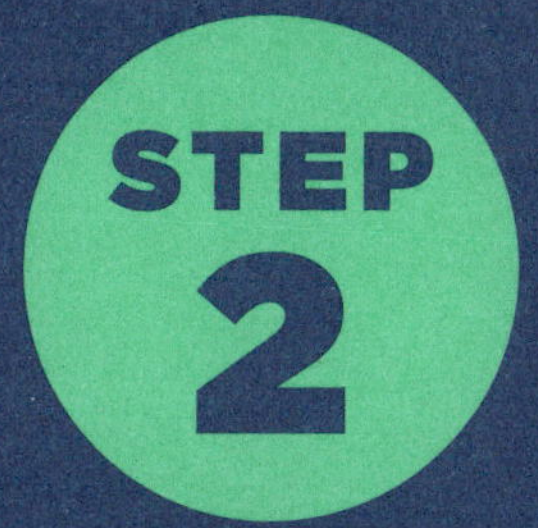

IDENTIFY YOUR TARGET

"Winter forms our character and brings out our best."

—TIM ALLEN

What do you want cold therapy to do for you? Now that you have a firm grip on the science and healing potential inherent in cold therapy, it's time to answer that question and define exactly what you want out of your practice.

Identifying your specific desired outcome is key. Giving cold therapy a try without a specific goal in mind is like plotting your course on a map without a destination. Yes, you'll wind up somewhere. But it's not likely to be where you hoped you'd find yourself.

Think of this step as a funnel. Over the course of this chapter, you'll be guided through the process of narrowing your goal or goals down to something more focused, a bullseye that allows for precise measurement and verification. That, in turn, will set you up for the future steps. It will lead you to the best possible cold therapy method for you and your health, allow you to measure results precisely, and give you useful insight into how to tweak your regimen to make it even more powerful.

To help you narrow down your thought process, the various objectives people traditionally hope to accomplish with cold therapy are broken down here one by one. Let's be clear, though. Health and wellness rarely relate to just one condition, disease, or ideal state. Most types of cold therapy will potentially affect more than one condition or health goal. You'll get the most out of your experience by considering how any potential goal you have dovetails with others. If you're hoping to achieve multiple benefits (e.g., boosting immunity and reducing mental stress or depression), create a priority list. The goal at the top will be the one you'll match to a particular method; the others will be used to measure success.

There's no law that says you must limit yourself to one cold therapy method just because it seems like the best way to address your primary goal. Stay open to potentially using more than one type, and certainly leave room for your personal preferences. For example, swimming in natural bodies of water only to get out and towel down on a rocky beach with a bracing wind in your face may not be your jam. Your situation is unique, so the best strategy for you is going to be unique as well.

With all that in mind, let's look at the goals that cold therapy is best equipped to address.

GOAL: HEAL INJURY OR TRAUMA

The human body breaks down in a remarkable number of ways. You can tweak your shoulder in a rough fender bender. An innocent game of pickup basketball can lead to painful ankle sprain. Or maybe a life of outdoor adventuring has led you to knee replacement surgery. The power of cold can improve all those cases of damage—and far more. In fact, accidental damage and trauma are conditions for which cutting edge cold-therapy technology is incredibly well-suited.

If your goal is to get back to your old self, moving around like normal, count yourself lucky. You've got a whole bunch of options from which to choose.

Trauma to a specific body part or area is usually treated with targeted cold therapy. This allows you to expose localized damaged tissue to the healing benefits of the therapy for much longer than you could reasonably maintain if your whole body was exposed. As a bonus, this type of technology allows you precision control over placement, time, and temperature.

The SMART Approach

Want to quickly and efficiently define the health goals you'd like to address with cold therapy? Take a page out of the professional management playbook. Since 1981, when management consultant and entrepreneur George Doran first proposed the system, the SMART method has been adopted by a variety of industries, from business to athletics to medicine. This is a straightforward and effective method for establishing verifiable and measurable goals, and can be a great way to ultimately determine how well your particular cold therapy is delivering against your expectations.

SMART is an acronym. It stands for:

SPECIFIC: "I want to limit pain and speed recovery in my leg muscles after a long bike ride every other day."

MEASURABLE: "Immediately post workout, waist-deep submersion in 50°F (10°C) water for two minutes. Goal is to reduce riding time over set distance by 5 percent in one month."

ACHIEVABLE: "As I become accustomed to the water temperature, I'll increase exposure by one minute each week. I'll measure riding time over distance during that first month."

RELEVANT: "I want to compete in a race in six months, meeting or beating my target time."

TIME LIMIT: "I'll do an in-depth assessment of my progress every two weeks, with a commitment to the current cold therapy regimen for at least six weeks."

Translating your experience to these types of data points means you won't rely on a gut feeling to determine if cold therapy is yielding the results you want. It's a concrete way to judge if you're getting any closer to your goal and will be essential for Step 5, when you begin refining your regimen.

SMART has helped dozens of companies and individuals hit their targets. It can be a great way for you to gauge success in your cold therapy journey.

ACCIDENTAL INJURY

The key to bouncing back from injuries small and large is to accelerate recovery and recuperation. That's where cold therapy shines.

Cold therapy has two potential and interrelated roles to play in injury treatment and healing. The first is the more immediate: reduce inflammation and cut down recovery time. The second is to dial back the pain during healing, so that you can rehab the area and get back to your normal movement and activity. Targeted localized cold therapy options often completely alleviate the need for other types of pain relief and makes rehabilitating and rejuvenating movement easier.

More modest injuries call for the most basic cold therapy—a cold compress, ice bag, or cold pad. Sometimes simple is best, and there is a reason these solutions have been around for millennia. Ideally, this type of cold therapy is part of a RICE (Rest, Ice, Compression, and Elevation) regimen. Localized cold should be applied for twenty minutes at a time as soon as possible after the injury, with a thirty-minute gap between applications, for the first forty-eight hours. After that, experts recommend that you switch to an application of heat if you still need relief.

POST-SURGERY HEALING

Cold therapy to aid post-surgery healing is a modern application, but one that has quickly proven its worth. A 2024 study measuring recovery and pain after breast cancer surgery found that the pace of healing was quicker and pain relief far greater in patients who integrated cold therapy into their recovery. Stunningly, only 4 percent of the targeted study participants needed additional pharmaceutical painkillers as opposed to 100 percent of the control group.

Post-surgical cold therapy will have the greatest impact in the first forty-eight hours after surgery. Beyond that window of opportunity, the healing benefits of cold exposure declines. In fact, after this initial phase, continued localized application of cold packs or cuffs may slow recovery because it will reduce blood flow and diminish nerve and hormone signals crucial to efficient healing. Regularly applying heat to the surgery site after

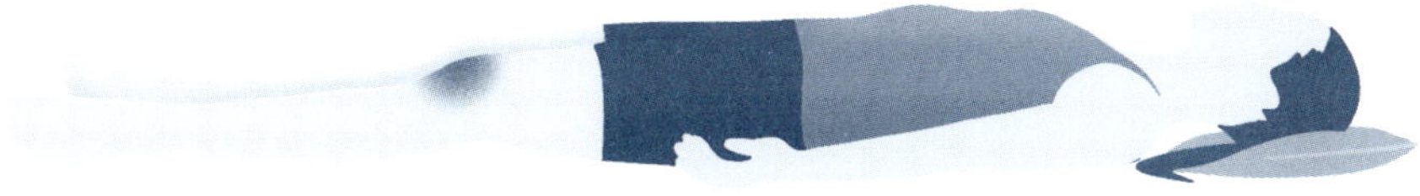

Rest

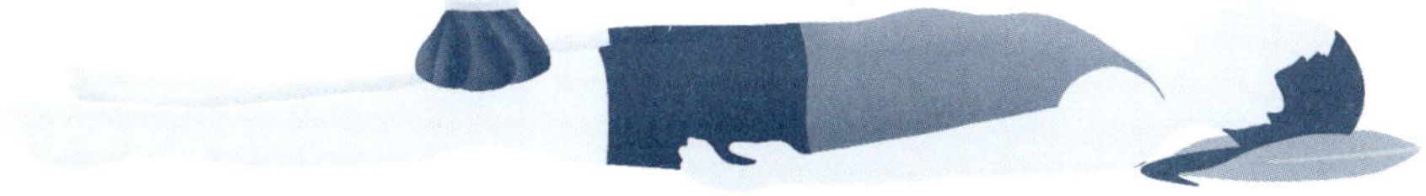

Ice

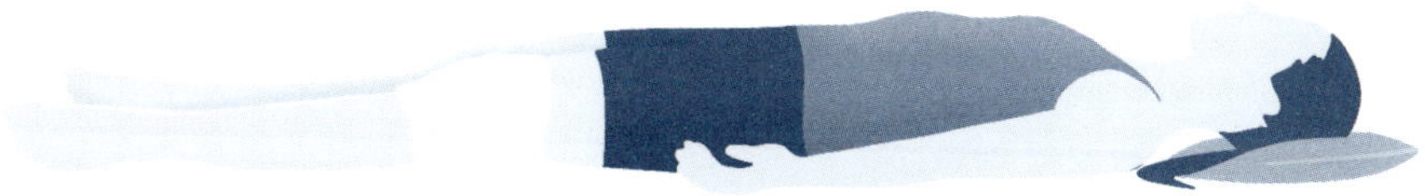

Compression

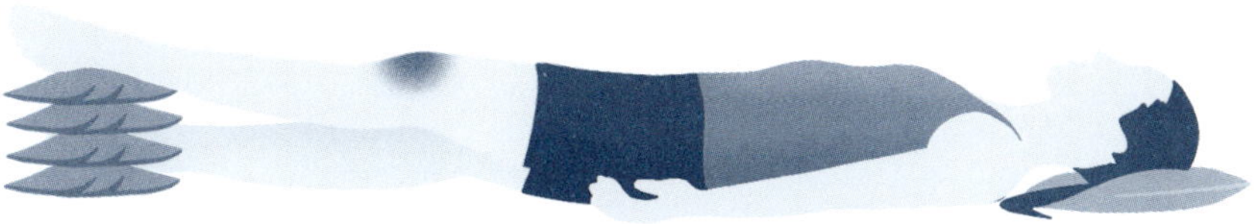

Elevation

that initial period will be the better strategy. The heat increases blood flow to the area, flooding it with nutrients and efficiently removing waste that is generated as the tissue repairs itself.

In any case, follow your care provider's guidance. Surgeons, especially, have deep experience optimizing low temperatures for post-surgical healing. The most common injuries and surgical repairs that leverage targeted cold therapy are damage to joints, including:

- Knee or hip replacement
- Wrist or elbow repair
- Shoulder reconstruction
- Lower back surgery
- Knee ACL, MCL, and meniscus surgery
- Broken ankle repair and stabilization

In all of these cases, manufacturers have developed wearable wraps that deliver cold at a consistent temperature over time. Although many are available direct to patients, it usually makes more sense to rent them through your care provider so that you can be reimbursed through insurance.

GOAL: REBOUND ATHLETICALLY

Many of the same principles that make cold therapy so effective for trauma healing make it just as promising to aid recovery from the damage caused by athletic exertion. Whereas injuries and most surgeries are unanticipated, damage from athletic exertion is a result of purposeful action. That means you can plan your recuperation and even use it to boost performance.

It's important to understand that the science around using cold therapy for athletic recovery and performance is evolving. Making things more complex, the therapy works differently from sport to sport and athlete to athlete. That shouldn't be surprising. The toll on a body from a long martial arts class is far different than the damage incurred by running a timed mile. Also, elite and professional athletes have been studied far more than have weekend warriors and other casual athletes. Regardless, the conclusions drawn from high-level athletes should translate down the skill ladder.

So far, athletic cold therapy has been focused on recovery from the tissue damage done during excessive exertion, with improvements to performance largely a consequence rather than primary focus. But boosting long-term performance may be the real prize of a long-term cold therapy regimen.

Athletes often turn to more than one type of cold therapy to achieve full recovery. Take a college or professional baseball pitcher, for example. The stress and strain of throwing eighty or ninety blisteringly fast pitches, with various arm angles and grips, translates to a lot of elbow and shoulder inflammation. Joint ice wraps are the most common treatment among amateurs and pros. Used immediately after pitching, this basic application relieves post-exertion joint pain and discomfort, substantially reduces inflammation, and speeds the return to action.

However, a pitcher doesn't just use (or overuse) their arm. Throwing a baseball again and again involves the entire body. In fact, the sport's insiders know from experience that every pitch is thrown from the legs first. So, any pitcher might well benefit from a plunge in a whole-body ice bath in addition to elbow and shoulder cold wraps.

The same is true of a club tennis player who hits the court four times a week and even enters the occasional amateur tournament. The elbow joint bears the most obvious strain. But given the amount of running, fast stops, and quick cuts that a competitive match entails, the tennis player, too, might benefit from localized cold therapy on the dominant elbow in combination with a whole-body ice bath or cryochamber session.

POST-WORKOUT THERAPY

Timing is key in using any cold therapy and no more so than in speeding recovery from athletic exertion. Research has shown, for instance, that a cold plunge is most effective when taken as soon after exercising as possible. The data suggests waiting will reduce the beneficial impact.

The time of day is no less important. In general, when it comes to cold therapy, morning is best. The mechanism of lowering internal temperature combined with the process of the body reheating after cold therapy mimics the circadian rhythm your nervous system follows throughout the day. Evening ice baths interrupt that pattern and have even been shown to disrupt sleep. However, every case is different. Athletes in general are best served by engaging in cold therapy right after their workout is over, at whatever time that may be.

The duration of any cold therapy is also an important factor—and one that will vary based on the type of therapy you've chosen. But in general, when using cold therapy for endurance recovery and performance the longer the exposure the better the performance boost. However, shorter duration at lower temperatures is best for recovery from high intensity interval training (HIIT).

You must also consider frequency. Practicing a cold therapy three times per week is the most common, although athletes who want to optimize benefits usually add cold therapy to the post-workout routine—often five times a week. You'll find specific recommendations for timing, duration, and scheduling in Step 4.

Not all types of cold therapy work equally as well in repairing what is known as "exercise-induced muscle damage" (EIMD)—the chief measure of athletic recovery. In fact, a 2020 study found that whole-body cryotherapy, using a cold-air cryochamber, was more effective at repairing damage than any type of cold-water therapy. While more research is needed, it is good to know that cold plunge baths are not your only option.

Research data aside, each athlete is different. That's why training regimens vary and workout trends come and go. Ultimately, getting to the ideal cold therapy practice that best complements your athletic pursuits will be a matter of balance existing science with personal preference and a little bit of experimentation.

WHO BENEFITS MOST?

As you might imagine, cold therapy is most useful for athletes who train and compete in hot weather or conditions, and those that follow a regular, hardcore training routine. Sports that involve challenges to the whole body, such as beach volleyball, tennis, baseball, and even bowling will likely realize a big benefit from a whole-body cold therapy regimen post-practice and after competitions.

The science behind cold therapy also means the practice is particularly effective for endurance athletes, such as long-distance runners, cyclists, and soccer players. Immersion in cold water, specifically, can reduce the immediate inflammation from overexertion of large muscles like the thighs and help flush waste products like lactic acid out of the muscles. This speeds recovery so that athletes can return to peak competition time and speed faster.

Research has shown the whole-body immersion cold therapy can be especially useful in recovery from HIIT. Less apparent, but no less important, is cold therapy's potential role in athletic injury performance. By quickly alleviating inflammation and stopping or reversing tissue damage, any cold therapy can be an excellent tool in potentially heading off overuse injuries, like tendonitis or strained muscles. While there is not a lot of research on the topic, the science points to that benefit.

But not every athlete may get quite as much from cold therapy, especially weight trainers, power lifters, and athletes who focus specifically on similar resistance exercise (pretty much anyone who is seeking what is called *hypertrophy*—the induced increase in size and mass of muscle). Because the protein synthesis and inflammation that occur right after lifting weights is a critical part of hypertrophy, these athletes are best served by waiting at least four hours after exercise to engage in cold therapy. At that point, they'll still realize some anti-inflammatory benefit.

Lastly, there is a less tangible upside that athletes can enjoy from regular cold therapy. Just as the effort to overcome physical challenges drives physical development in skills, strength, and endurance, the mental challenge

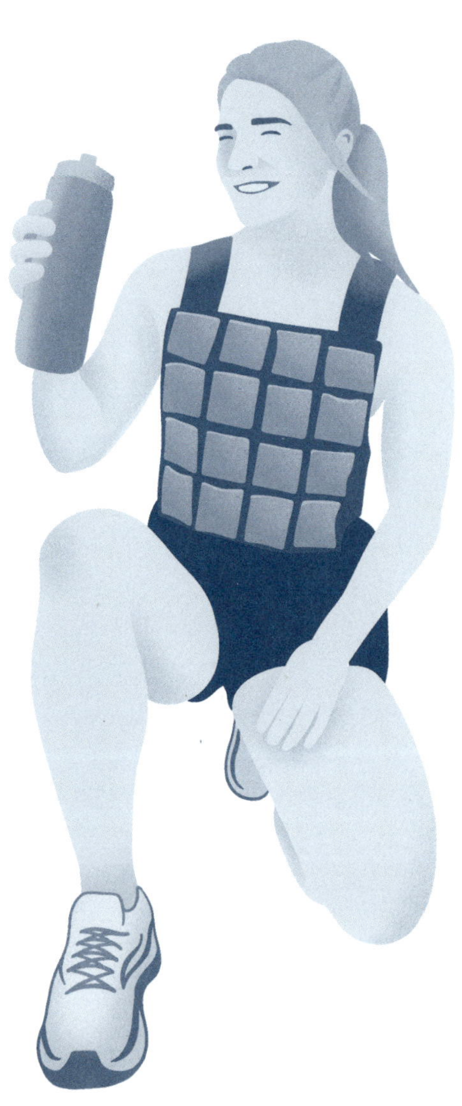

The Cold Start

Any endurance activity or strenuous exercise causes the body's internal engine to heat up. The quicker your internal temperature rises, the faster your body will hit the wall of fatigue and exhaustion. Dehydration causes your cells to produce energy less efficiently. Lactic acid and other waste products build up in muscle tissue as the body overheats. A rising internal temperature does the athlete no favors. Unfortunately, heat is a natural result of exertion.

Advocates and researchers are increasingly taking a novel approach to that biological reality: Begin any athletic exertion with a lower internal temperature.

By cooling the body *before* you start exercising, your system will theoretically take longer to overheat to exhaustion. That's the fundamental assumption behind the theory of "pre-cooling," an unusual offshoot of traditional cold therapy.

The main types of pre-cooling methods that have been tried include cold water immersion, consuming ice, wearing cooling garments such as a pre-frozen vest like the illustration on the left, or mittens and whole-body cryotherapy (air cooling).

A 2012 clinical analysis analyzed prior studies to determine which of the first three were most effective. Researchers found that cold water immersion appears to hold the most significant potential for increasing endurance and performance levels.

Available research data also indicates that the athletes who are likeliest to benefit from pre-cooling are resistance exercise competitors or anyone building muscle mass, those who hope to increase mental focus and alertness, and others who are concerned about overheating during longer sporting events.

Embracing pre-cooling will likely come down to how avid an athlete you are (translating to how willing you are to go to extremes for relatively modest performance gains), and personal preferences. Many people simply wouldn't embrace the idea of a cold plunge or wearing an ice-cold vest before their five-mile (8 km) run or stationary cycle workout.

However, if you're open to experimenting and willing to undergo the discomfort, preliminary evidence suggests that a pre-exercise ice bath or cold-water swim for three to ten minutes might measurably boost your training time and the effectiveness of any endurance workout.

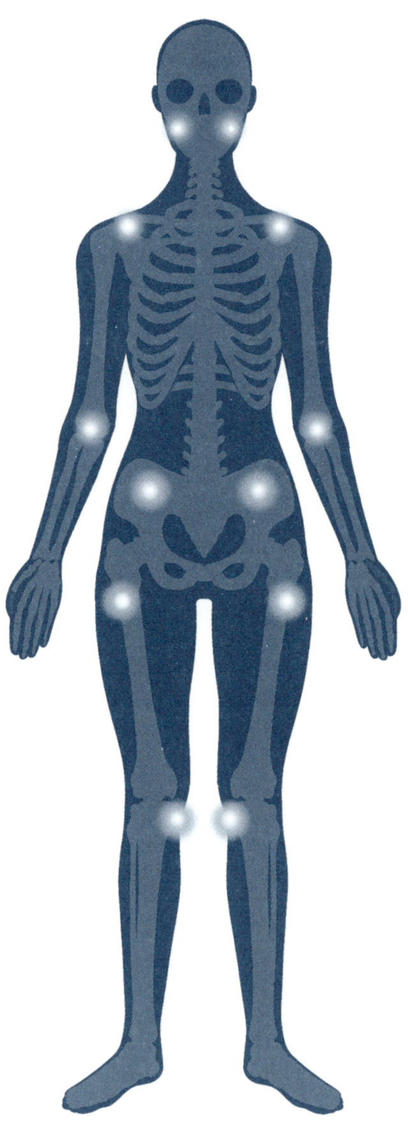

Fibromyalgia, like many autoimmune diseases, causes multiple points of chronic pain and inflammation. Whole-body cold therapy is usually much more effective than targeted types.

inherent in enduring a set period in cold temperature builds strong will and can help athletes overcome the psychological roadblocks they encounter. Some studies suggest cold therapy improves mental outlook, attitude, and mood. And while those are hard to measure in terms of athletic performance, few athletes would discount the fact that mental condition and a positive focus play crucial roles in athletic achievement.

GOAL: FIGHT DISEASE

Cold therapy combats disease on two fronts. First, it diminishes the inflammation that drives illnesses from arthritis to inflammatory bowel disease (IBD) and Crohn's disease to chronic obstructive pulmonary disease (COPD) and lupus. It is, in fact, an especially powerful tool in dealing with chronic inflammatory conditions, like fibromyalgia.

Second, but no less important, cold therapy eases pain. Anyone who is dealing with long-term back pain from a deteriorating disc or the ever-present ache of osteoarthritis can attest to how essential pain relief is in treating any disease. It's one thing to have your mobility curtailed, but overwhelming pain on a daily basis can quickly decimate quality of life and is an absolute joy killer. It also makes any productive physical rehabilitation much more difficult.

The problem is that discomfort is built into any disease, and managing chronic disease is a challenge. The idea of subjecting yourself to even more discomfort with a cold plunge or sitting in a cryochamber can be unappealing at best. In many cases, patients will find it easiest to slowly introduce cold therapy into their disease treatment plan. Once the benefits become apparent, there is a more obvious carrot at the end of the metaphorical stick, often making it mentally easier to integrate longer and more intense exposures or more frequent cold therapy sessions.

There are also much more specialized types of cold therapy focused on one disease. The most interesting of these is *cryoimmunotherapy*. This cancer treatment pairs directly freezing tumor cells in a process known *cryoablation* with targeted immunotherapy. The former kills cancer cells, triggering a response that is amplified by the latter. Cryoimmunotherapy is not right for every cancer, but it can be an effective treatment option in certain cases.

It bears repeating here that cold therapy isn't right for treating all diseases and conditions. Specifically, cold therapy should not be used to treat heart disease or any condition that involves circulatory problems. Given the underlying mechanism, the therapy will be most effective for conditions in which inflammation is a significant contributing factor or a primary symptom.

All that aside, the best way to treat a disease is to prevent it in the first place. There is some evidence to suggest cold therapy can, as a part of a healthy lifestyle, play a role in disease prevention. However, there is far less clinical evidence supporting this role because prevention is incredibly difficult to study.

WHAT AILS YOU?

Certain illnesses are particularly good targets for treatment with cold therapy. These include:

Autoimmune diseases: Diseases such as fibromyalgia, lupus, multiple sclerosis, inflammatory bowel disease, and rheumatoid arthritis are all very different but share two important factors: exceptional systemic neurological inflammation and an immune system response that mistakes the body's own tissues for foreign invaders. They also share something else: profound and long-term pain. Studies show that cold therapy can have some level of positive impact on all those aspects of autoimmune diseases.

Most obviously, whole-body cold exposure will diminish both the pain of the disease and the inflammation causing the pain. There is also evidence that systemic exposure to significant cold can reduce the reaction of cytokines, protein molecules responsible for signaling cells to react to an immune system threat. The mood-boosting effects of repeated cold exposure can also be a big plus for people suffering under the frustratingly persistent symptoms of their body attacking itself. People with autoimmune diseases often also deal with some level of depression or anxiety.

Prediabetes and diabetes: Research has shown that repeated cold exposure can improve what is known as "glucose metabolism," the process by which the body removes sugar from the bloodstream. Repeated cold exposure also elevates levels of a protein that aids in removing glucose from the bloodstream. These conclusions point to the role a cold therapy regimen could play in potentially helping to prevent type 2 diabetes when someone is diagnosed with prediabetes, as well as to its potential to moderate the impact of type 2 diabetes in concert with other lifestyle changes.

Migraines and other headaches: Although there is not yet significant evidence that whole-body exposure to cold will impact the intensity, frequency, or duration of migraines, ample evidence shows that direct cold application to the neck and head for at least twenty minutes can have a significant impact on reducing the crippling pain of this condition. Further research is in the pipeline.

GOAL: CHILL OUT CHRONIC CONDITIONS

Whether persistent damage was caused by an accident or illness, pain is the most debilitating hallmark of chronic conditions. Consider the incredibly common and often mysterious back injury. Because the spine, back nerves, and related musculature are so complicated, even talented surgeons struggle to repair—much less reverse—serious damage to the back. More often than not, back injuries or structural defects are both chronic and degenerative. They limit mobility and create pain that is exacerbated by any bodily movement. The immobility and pain can be overwhelming and life-disrupting.

Medical professionals often turn to powerful drugs to help patients with back pain. But, as the opioid crisis in America proves, pain relief drugs have a huge downside and may not be a healthy or sustainable long-term pain management strategy in and of themselves. Cold therapy can be just as good at numbing nerve receptors, dulling and even eliminating chronic pain. This is true not only in the moment but for a significant period of time after the sufferer ends the cold therapy session.

As pain eases, the sufferer can move around more easily, which further aids healing and back health (not to mention quality of life). Diminished pain can, for instance, allow back patients to pursue restorative physical rehab exercises.

Different types of cold therapy can offer even more benefits for anyone managing chronic injuries. Cold swims not only ease the pain from a damaged back, hip, knee, or shoulder, but also the water is uniquely suited to support joints and skeletal structure in a way no other medium can. Swimming is a safe way to engage in a beneficial motion that will help rehab a damaged joint or problem area such as a damaged lower back. And, of course, the widely reported euphoric feeling may combat the depression that so commonly accompanies long-term chronic pain—especially the back pain that limits both movement and living your life.

GOAL: TURBOCHARGE THE IMMUNE SYSTEM

You don't have to have a disease or trauma to benefit from cold therapy. In fact, the potential for cold therapy to improve immune system function may be one of its most important functions. Maybe you're trying to head off a yearly bout of flu or recurrent sicknesses you pick up by way of your child's daycare. Perhaps you want to ensure the best protection possible against the genetic diseases that run in your family. Whatever the case, the relationship between cold and immune system response has been investigated for decades. There is a good chance that if boosting your immune system is a primary health goal, cold therapy can be an incredibly powerful tool in your arsenal.

The idea isn't new. Advocates have long promoted regular cold showers or ice baths as a simple, effective to way to boost immune system response. A good amount of science backs that up.

All the way back in 1996, researchers found that regular cold-water immersion measurably improved the number of disease-fighting T-cells, monocytes, cancer-fighting natural killer cells, and other helper cells circulating in young, healthy, male test subjects. The effect became more pronounced over time (the study followed subjects through three cold therapy sessions per week for six weeks). It's important to note that it took time and exposure to build a robust immune system response.

Other studies have found cold water swimmers enjoy better protection against respiratory infections, an increase in antioxidant factors in the blood, and a greater number of specific immune response cells like natural killer cells. The response relates to how our bodies process healthy stress. When you put the right amount of resistance stress on bones, for instance, the bones uptake more calcium and become stronger. As we challenge our physiological systems under the adverse conditions of extreme cold, it's not surprising that the body's immune system answers the call by dialing up the proliferation of blood-borne protector cells. (You'll find more about adaptive stress response [hormesis] on page 29.)

If improving your immune system is your goal, however, keep this in mind: No single wellness practice is the magic bullet of immunity. Cold therapy's effect on your immune system will be most robust when it's coupled with other immune-boosting lifestyle practices, like good sleep hygiene and habits, a healthy diet, and stress-reduction practices like socializing and meditation.

GOAL: MANAGE MENTAL WELL-BEING

You won't find many cold therapy advocates or enthusiasts who don't sing the praises of the practice for improving mood and creating a general feeling of well-being. That common anecdotal experience reveals the potential for cold beyond the physical. Mental health professionals and patients alike are understandably excited at the prospect of cold therapy controlling—or even reversing—the life-disrupting effects of diseases such as depression and anxiety.

The idea of cold therapy reducing or even replacing the need for powerful psychiatric medications is especially exciting, given that those drugs and therapies can be unpredictable and often include severe side effects.

Existing research just scratches the surface. Mental health and mental disease are areas that are notoriously difficult to clinically study. The research that is available is often restricted in sample size. For instance, a widely cited 2018 study followed the progress of a young woman with major depressive disorder and anxiety. She was able to discontinue her drug regimen thanks to a regular schedule of open-water cold swims.

However, studies like this, along with what we already know about the science of cold therapy, give us a glimpse into the practice's promise in aiding mental health and mental disease management and recovery. Enduring cold therapy is a way of managing a certain type of stress (that has both a mental and physical component). As you become more accustomed to cold therapy, you improve your ability to effectively handle other types of stress in your life. This is what's known as *cross adaption*.

And cold therapy isn't exactly new territory for the mental health community. Sanitariums have, over the last two centuries, regularly turned to cold plunges as a treatment for depression and other conditions in different time periods (what was called *hysteria*).

The science supports this application. As described above, cold immersion and exposure spur the release of a number of hormones, including powerful hormones like dopamine and endorphins that regulate mood. These can have an outsized impact on depression and other mental health issues. The boost in endorphin levels alone can counter the symptoms of mild depression and anxiety. One recent study found that participants experienced a substantial improvement in mood after a single cold plunge. Cold showers seem to have a less powerful but similar effect, although cold showers are studied much less than any other cold therapy.

Depression and anxiety: A 2023 study found that participants were more positive and less nervous after a cold water plunge. The researchers attributed this to connections between areas of the brain responsible for focus, emotions, and self-control. Another white paper used the science of cold stress as a basis to postulate that cold showers could offer a simple, low-impact treatment for clinical depression. This is not to say that cold therapy can or should be the sole treatment of, or considered a cure for, clinical depression or anxiety. However, the science seems to indicate that regular cold therapy has a role to play in treating those conditions and can potentially have a significant impact.

PTSD: A groundbreaking and ongoing study out of Swansea University is currently exploring the usefulness of cold therapy as a potential element in the treatment for post-traumatic stress disorder (PTSD). Initial findings are positive, showing improvement among test subjects. This will likely inspire further studies into this incredibly important subject. However, before the study's completion and publication, anyone wrestling with the devastating effects of PTSD or similar syndromes can experiment with cold therapy with little risk (unless it's triggering to the person's particular condition).

Addiction: It's a fact that cold therapy elevates the "feel-good" hormone dopamine and the body's own pleasure-promoting endorphins that help combat cravings. Depending on the type of cold therapy, the duration of the practice, and other specifics, those higher levels may last for hours or longer. Cold therapy also appears to calm and help mediate the part of the brain responsible for self-control. Taken together, these facts may well demonstrate the usefulness of cold therapy as a simple and beneficial element in the treatment of alcoholism, drug addiction, and other addictions.

GOAL: SUPPORT OR PROMOTE WEIGHT LOSS

It might seem like a bit of stretch, but cold therapy can play a part in weight reduction. Exposure to cold air or frigid water triggers the release of the hormone noradrenaline, which floods white fat cells. That causes those cells to convert to much more efficient beige and brown fat cells. Brown fat is commonly known as brown adipose tissue (BAT).

Seems like one type of fat would be the same as any other, right? Wrong. Beige and brown fat, like white fat, get their unimaginative names from their actual colors. Under a microscope, the fat cells appear either dark

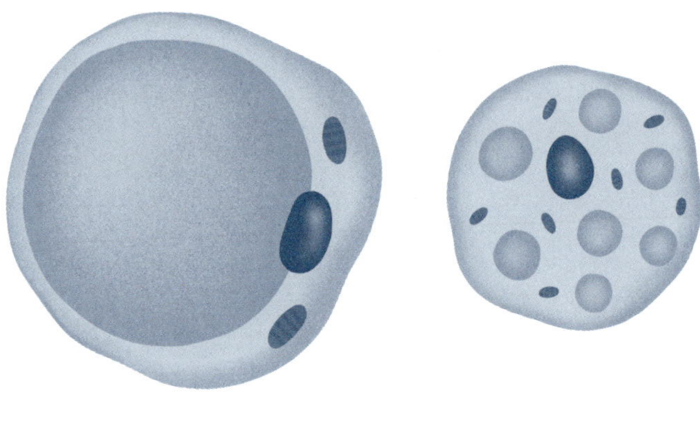

A Large White Fat Cell A Smaller Brown Fat Cell

beige or brown due to a high density of mitochondria, those cellular energy engines. That density is what makes brown fat so very different—and plainly more desirable from a health point of view—from white fat.

The good news is that brown fat is much more active than other types. The more brown fat you have than white fat, the more calories your body will naturally burn throughout the course of the day.

What's more, research has revealed that when brown fat is activated during cold therapy, it rapidly burns calories to heat the body (a process called *non-shivering thermogenesis*). In the moment, this speeds up metabolism and lasts as long as the body combats the effects of extreme low temperature.

But there's more. Brown fat is the health gift that keeps on giving. Studies in mice have found that brown adipose tissue is integral in improving insulin sensitivity and regulating blood glucose levels. This speaks to its potential role in lowering the risk of diabetes even as it burns calories. The effect appears to persist even long after you return to a warm room or car.

The more frequent the exposure to cold, the more robust the brown fat reaction and amped-up calorie burning. The body, in turn, builds stores of high-energy brown fat, putting less emphasis on reserving calories in the more common white fat.

There is not yet a programmatic approach to using cold therapy specifically for weight loss, but research continues, and the science indicates that this goal is well within the wheelhouse of the therapy's potential benefits. This presents the enticing possibility that simple and cheap cold therapy might be a substitute for expensive and disruptive semaglutide weight-loss drugs.

GOAL: IMPROVE SKIN HEALTH

It doesn't matter whether you're more concerned about keeping your body's largest organ in the peak of health and preventing conditions like eczema flare-ups or skin cancer, or are focused on creating the luxurious, beautiful glow that healthy, wrinkle-free skin has. Skin health should be a universal concern (and skin beauty and well-being are inextricably intertwined in any case).

Your skin is your largest organ, and keeping it healthy is as important as taking care of your other organs. Fortunately, cold therapy has been shown to offer benefits for both how your skin looks and how healthy it actually is. Controlled exposure to cold diminishes the inflammation that contributes to skin conditions from eczema to allergic dermatitis. That puffiness under your eyes and around your face when you haven't slept enough or drank too much is just inflammation by another name.

Cold strategically applied can tighten pores and skin structure, minimize wrinkling, help flush contaminants and waste products out of skin cells, increase healthy circulation, and more. A 2015 study found that targeted therapy to reduce wrinkling was effective without the potentially toxic side effects of biological or chemical treatments.

You'll discover more about specific routines that can aid your skin on page 80. But suffice it to say that cold therapy holds a lot of promise for both skin problems and general skin health—and will improve the way your skin looks, as a bonus.

GOAL: INCREASE LONGEVITY

Longevity is usually not a primary goal for people interested in cold therapy, but it's the rare person who doesn't hold this as at least a secondary goal to every other step they take in improving their health.

That's only natural. After all, what are you getting healthy for, if not to live a long and full life? Just as important, though, is staying healthy as long as you live. Nobody wants to spend the last decade of life immobile, suffering pain, and struggling with deteriorating health.

Cold therapy can theoretically help you live longer and healthier. There isn't a large body of research behind this (imagine how difficult it is to follow test subjects over the course of their lifespan—which is why research so far has been limited to small, short-lived organisms), but the science supports the idea.

Consider the process of *hormesis* (previously discussed on page 29). The more you bolster your body and mind's adaptive stress response, the less impact stress throughout your life will have on your well-being. Because we know that stress exacerbates almost every disease and can actually trigger some conditions, it's reasonable to assume this one effect of cold therapy can boost lifespan (and "healthspan"—how long you live in good health).

As we've seen, cold therapy also results in a proliferation of, and greater activity among, the mitochondria responsible for cellular energy production. More efficient cell activity translates to a longer life. The same is true when you improve immune system response and reduce inflammation throughout the body on an ongoing basis. Of course, both of those are well-chronicled results of a cold therapy regimen.

Lastly, there is substantial evidence that cold therapy boosts the production of antioxidants in your bloodstream, which work to protect cells from damage. The logical assumption is that cold therapy is most likely to impact longevity as a long-term and possibly lifelong practice.

Obviously, there are a great many potential applications for cold therapy. Your specific goals will depend on your own health situation, preferences, and desires. That doesn't mean that you are limited to one. Given the range of benefits cold therapy offers, you might choose to structure a regimen that addresses more than one goal.

In any case, make it formal. Write down your goals, define your baseline, and note benchmarks by which you can measure your success. Once you've clearly established where you want to go on this health journey, the next step is to choose a method for getting there.

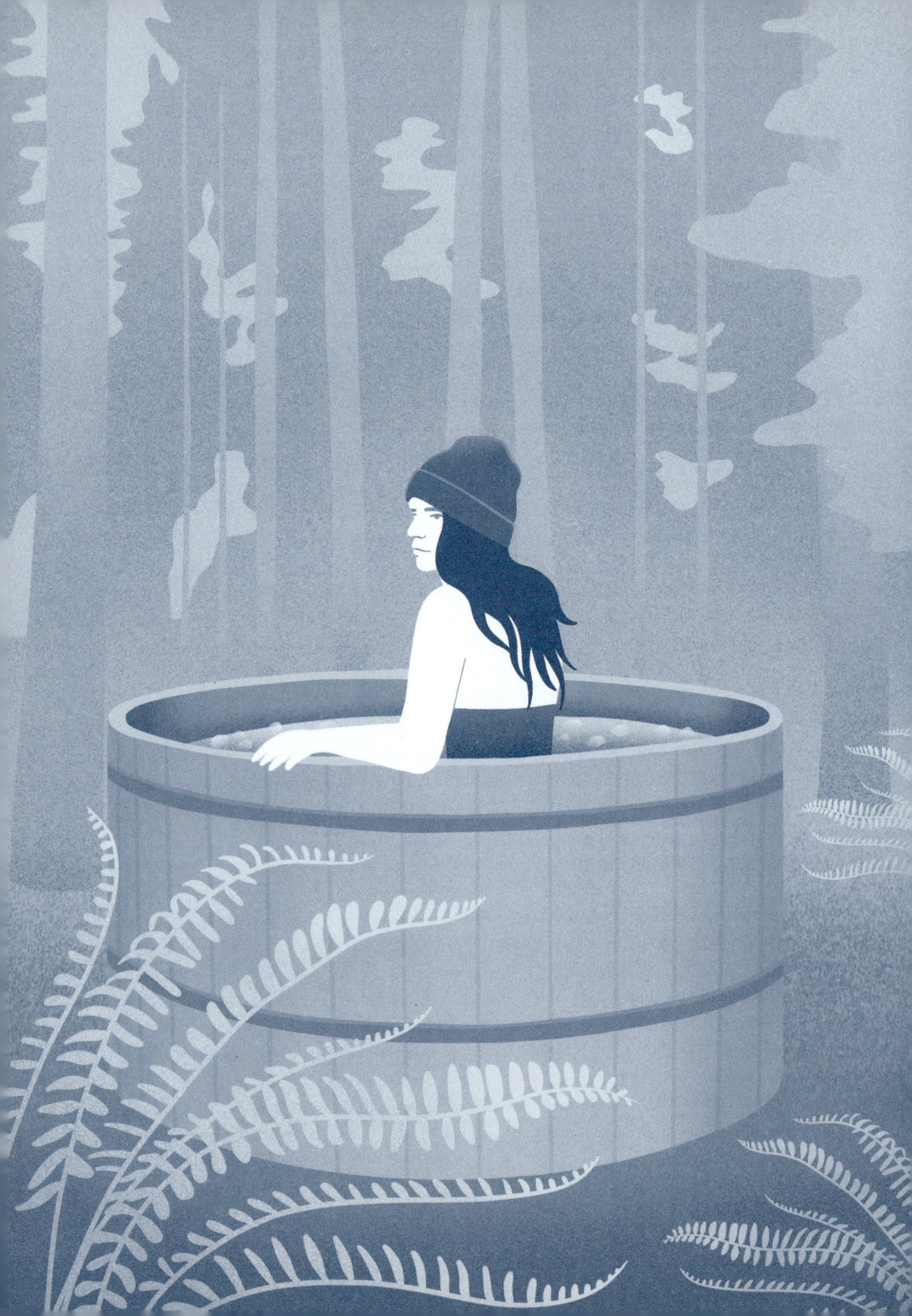

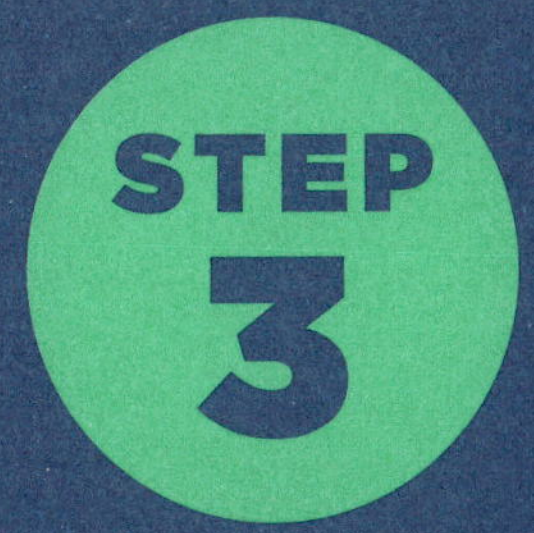

PICK YOUR PRACTICE

"To appreciate the beauty of a snowflake it is necessary to stand out in the cold."

—ARISTOTLE

Now that you've identified your health and wellness goals, it's relatively easy to select your cold therapy method of choice. That's what Step 3 is all about. As you read through this chapter, the method that is best for you will likely become apparent. But keep in mind that personal preference is just one part of picking your method; practicality also plays a part. For instance, while an ice bath plunge may achieve your goals quickly, it may simply be unendurable for you personally, and a cold shower may be more practical.

That's okay. Choices abound—and your method of choice can change, too, as your endurance and comfort level increases over time. You may find that you can eventually graduate to types of cold exposure that seemed impossible before. Keep an open mind.

Part of cold therapy is about intentionally guiding your own process. That's control under another name. When you control your own health journey, you're empowered and more likely to get to a good place of maximum health and well-being. Cold therapy is no more nor less than a tool. Be intentional and thoughtful in selecting a method, so that you can stick with the regimen as long as possible and realize substantial and lasting benefits.

These methods can be crudely broken down into two major categories that we've briefly touched on previously: targeted and whole body. Beyond those fundamental divisions, there is a lot of room to tailor the experience and adjust your method for just how much discomfort you're willing to endure. Let's start with targeted exposure.

STAY ON TARGET

Targeted, or "focused," cold therapy involves applying cold to one specific area of the body. The most basic and common form is an ice pack. It's also the simplest cold therapy. Unlike other therapy options, though, ice packs are short term and temporary. They are used to treat accidental trauma for the first forty-eight hours after the injury. They can also mitigate some of the pain of migraines and other chronic conditions, but are not highly effective in reducing chronic pain over the long term.

It's a case of a one-size-fits-all solution not serving any individual as efficiently as possible. Fortunately, there are many other targeted cold therapies that offer more powerful effects.

CUSTOM-MADE CHILL

Researchers and manufacturers continue to explore and exploit the power of cold to treat specific areas of the body and unique situations. If your goal is to heal from shoulder surgery as quickly as possible or alleviate the pain and immobility of rheumatoid arthritis in your wrist, the following options are well worth exploring.

Cuffs, casts, and wraps: Undergoing surgery? Adjustable slip-on or strap-on wrap coverings connected to a cold-water pump are incredibly precise ways to speed healing and drastically reduce post-operative pain. These are normally rented from a medical supply house through your practitioner and rolled into the overall bill submitted to your insurance. However, they can also be purchased directly from several sources. Regardless, the idea is to circulate cold water around the damaged area for specific periods of

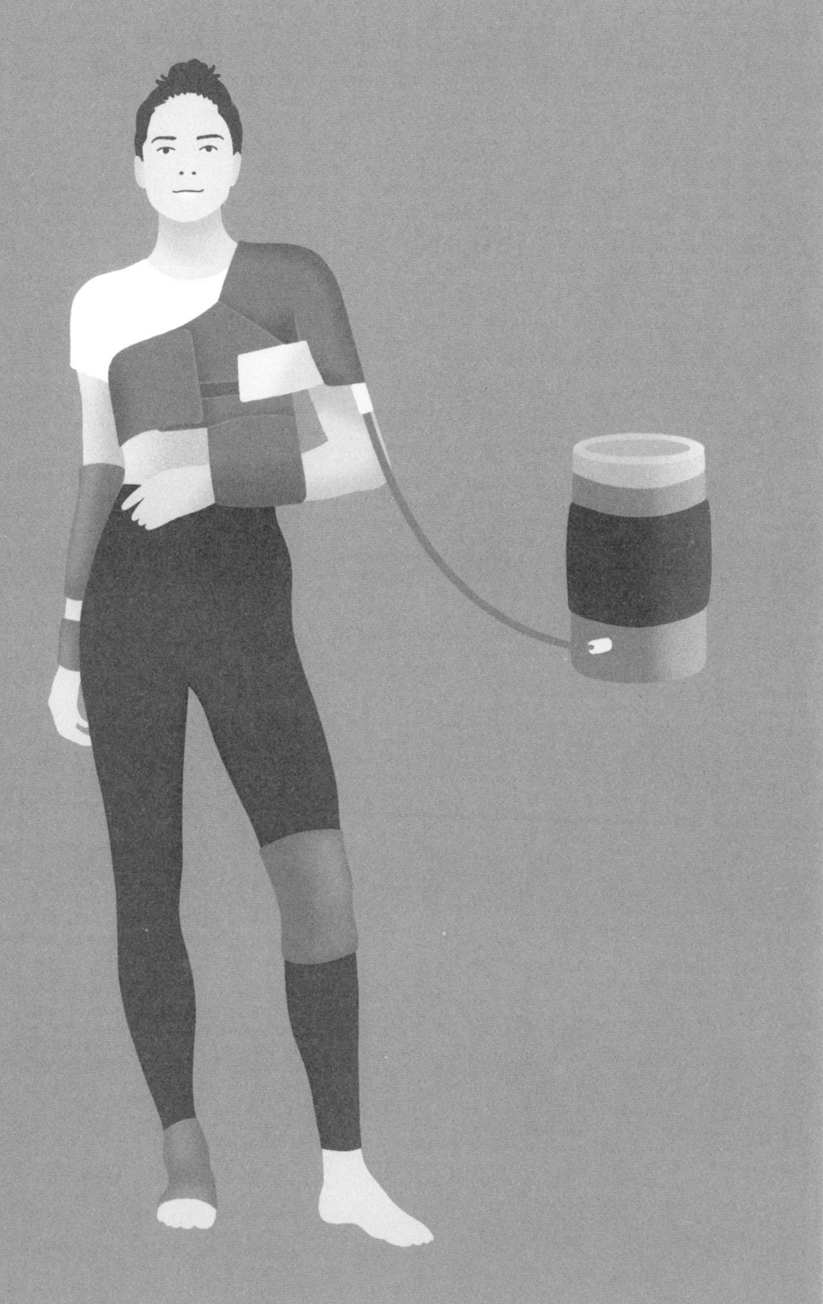

time. These wearables are usually used for the first few days of healing, after which physical therapy and heating pads take over.

Their usefulness is not, however, limited to surgical trauma. Cuffs, casts, and sleeves are all ideally suited to treating joints or limbs that have been injured or are affected by a chronic condition. You also don't need a surgeon or medical professional to prescribe one. More basic products using the same method include ice-water cooling chambers connected to flexible pads that can be used on any part of the body. The beauty of all these innovative devices is precision delivery of cold to exactly where it's needed.

Cold therapy wearables: These are simpler versions of pump-connected wraps, slings, and casts that require no machinery—making them less-expensive targeted therapy options. Examples include wearable cooling vests, chilled compression leg and arm sleeves, and compression joint sleeves. They are either kept in the freezer between uses or designed with pockets that hold gel packs that can be frozen and reused.

Although specific wearables like these can be used to treat chronic pain and inflammation, they are more often leveraged for athletic recovery. They are relatively inexpensive in relation to any pump-connected garment, making them an attractive option for athletes looking to explore how well cold therapy might serve them to recover from exertion.

FREEZING FOR BEAUTY

Another possible application for targeted cold exposure is in the world of beauty. Cold is increasingly being used for targeted beauty treatments. The potential is exceptional, because the therapy potentially offers an alternative to expensive creams, treatments like Botox, and other more drastic procedures like chemical peels. The most common cold therapy beauty treatment offered today is liquid nitrogen facials. Extremely cold liquid nitrogen vapor is carefully dispersed all over the face and neck to increase collagen production.

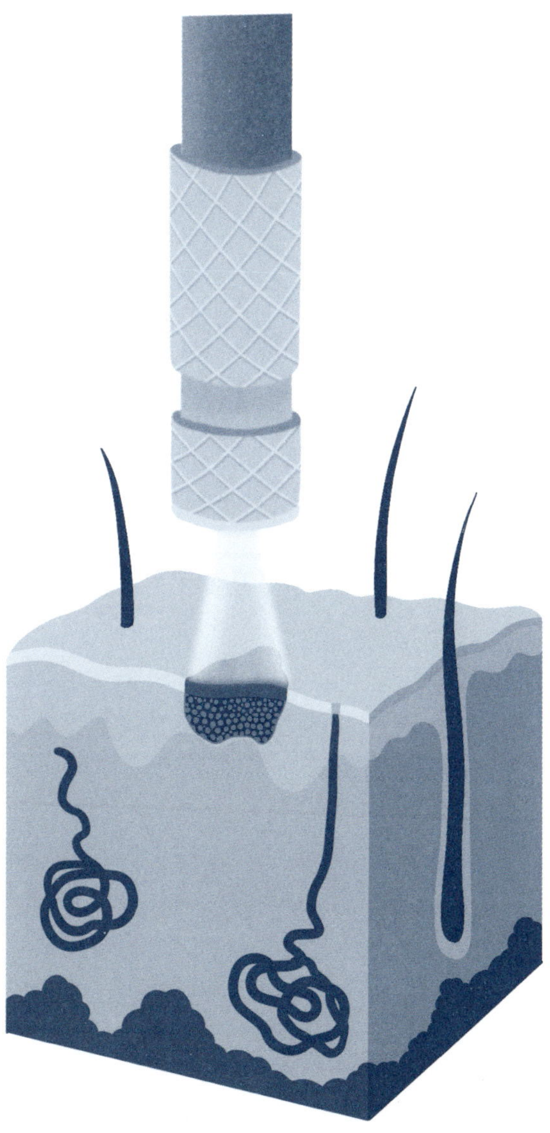

Dermatologists often use a directed spray of liquid nitrogen to kill abnormal skin growths and lesions. They, and plastic surgeons, use a cotton-wrapped wand to apply liquid nitrogen vapor all over the face and neck, which enhances collagen production and creates a healthier, more radiant skin tone.

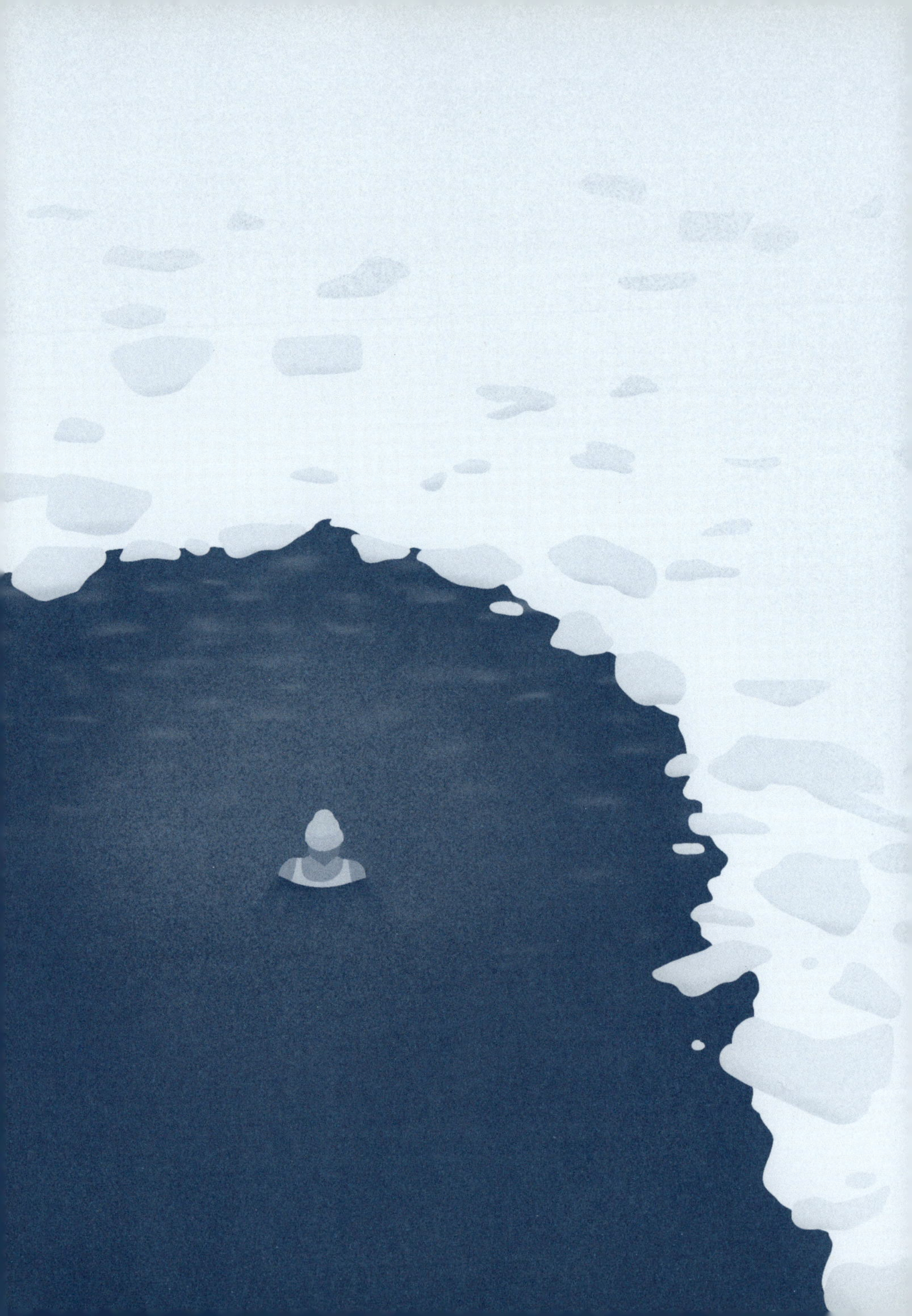

The treatment must be done by a qualified and experienced practitioner taking safety precautions (liquid nitrogen is capable of quickly causing frostbite and skin damage) but is quick and effective. The result is a refreshed appearance with glowing skin and diminished wrinkles.

If your personal goals revolve around dermatology or skincare, you might want to research the difference between cryotherapy and cold therapy. Dermatological cryotherapy is normally a surgical alternative in which focused sub-zero cold is used to destroy and remove irregular tissue like warts, lesions, and some tumors. Cryotherapy is a powerful and important tool in skin health, but it is not cold therapy as defined within the scope of this book.

TAKE IN THE WATERS

There are two kinds of whole-body immersion: cold water immersion and cold air exposure. As we covered in Step 1, each has its own benefits and drawbacks, and which one works best for you will largely depend on your lifestyle, goals, and personal preferences. You can think of cold water immersion as the classic method (cold air is a more recent innovation), and it is generally more accessible for most people. You can access it either in the wild, or—and this may be easier to begin with—in the comfort of your own home.

COLD WATER IMMERSION AT HOME

The simplest forms of cold therapy whole-body immersion are waiting for you in your bathroom. Cold showers and baths are the most basic ways to deliberately expose yourself to cold in a safe environment. The ease of use and control are why many advocates recommend that beginners start their journeys by exploring cold therapy with these methods.

Showers: Showers, in particular, are excellent cold therapy stepping stones. Showers are an easy way to determine how well you can adapt to cold exposure and to build up your tolerance. And as simple as they are, they can

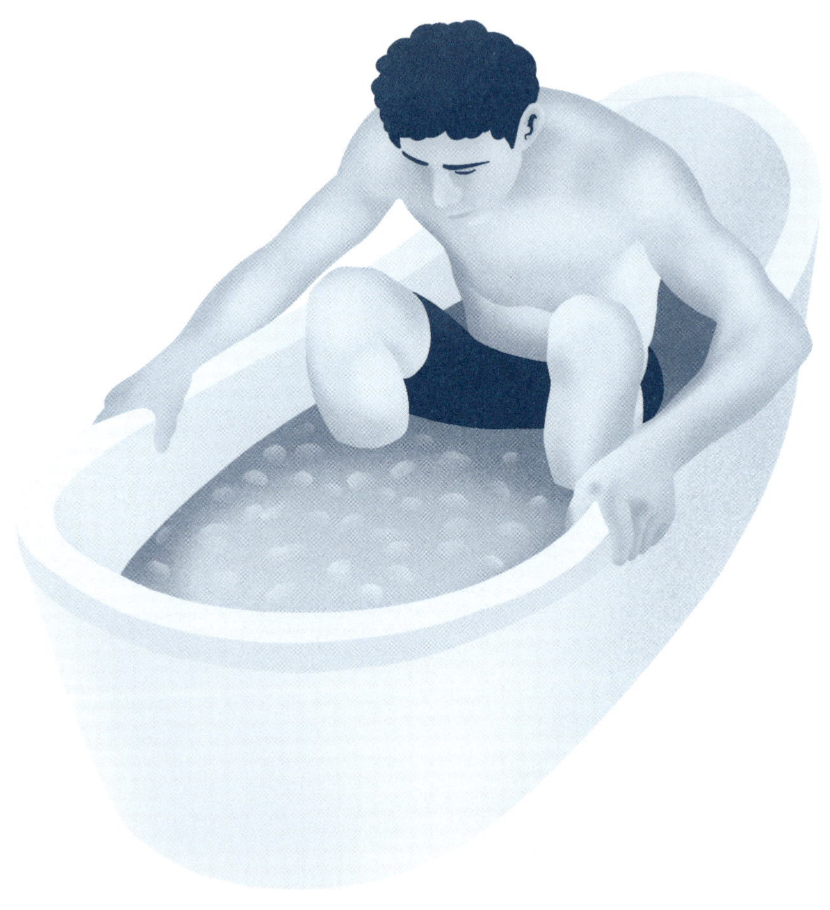

The simplest way to do an ice bath at home
is to simply fill your tub with ice cubes.

have a measurable impact on health. In fact, research has shown regular cold showers can boost the production of beneficial immune response cells. On a more superficial level, most people find cold showers easier to control, because they can choose what part of the body is exposed at any one time. Note, however, the effects of a cold shower are not as profound as other types of cold therapy—especially for goals like athletic recovery. Showers also do not appear to have as many health benefits as whole-body immersion in a cold-water bath.

Baths: Obviously, total immersion in a tub translates to more surface area chilled in a uniform way (unlike in a shower, where a large percentage of your body will always be out of a shower's spray at any given moment). An icy bath reduces your body's core temperature more quickly and efficiently, and improves circulation more comprehensively. That translates to significantly better muscle-strain recovery and general health benefits.

But note that not all ice baths are created equal. The most basic, of course, is simply filling your existing bathtub with cold water or a mix of water and ice. Depending on your tub size, the experience may or may not allow for total immersion. Your knees may stick up or most of your torso could be outside the water. To get maximum immersion in a home tub, you must be completely or mostly horizontal.

Cold bath advocates and experts consider a vertical position superior to a horizontal pose, because it affords the user much more control, and it is easier to breathe when sitting up or standing. Unimpeded breathing is crucial for most people to tolerate immersion to the target time.

Inflatables: Short of swapping out your current bathtub, you can upgrade to an inflatable cold therapy tub. These are relatively inexpensive and easy to use. However, they are also less durable, are prone to leaks, and are an extremely basic experience. They are a good choice for anyone who wants to try cold therapy but isn't certain they will stick with it over the long term.

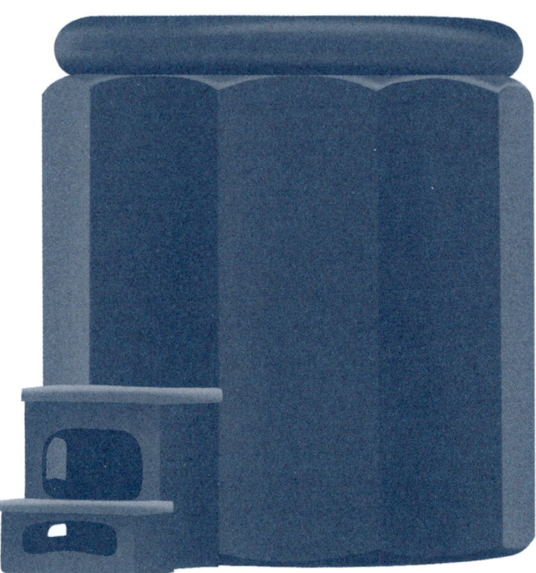

A commercial plunge tub can be a worthy investment as it gives you greater control over the temperature and includes other luxury features.

Freestanding cold plunge tanks or baths: Avid cold therapy proponents who have established a disciplined and regular schedule of several plunges per week may want to consider a more upscale option. Freestanding cold plunge tanks or baths are not inexpensive, but they offer a range of options that can amplify your cold therapy experience. They are insulated to retain precise temperatures longer and often include luxury options like state-of-the-art water filtration, onboard icemakers, nonslip surfaces, comfortable seating, LED readout screens, and even Wi-Fi compatibility. They are also distinctively styled to be eye-catching additions to any patio or outdoor area.

Be aware that plunge tubs require maintenance. They need to be regularly emptied and sanitized, and you should cover them whenever they're not in use (this is why it's good to buy one with a tight-fitting lid). It's important to follow the manufacturer's directions for use to the letter to avoid infections and malfunctions.

Even if one of these models is out of your price range you may be able to use one at your local gym. Increasingly, high-end gyms and clinics offer fully featured plunge tubs and reclining ice baths.

NATURE'S WHOLE-BODY IMMERSION EXPERIENCES

An ice bath or plunge requires both a single-minded focus and tolerance to discomfort. Sitting in a tub doing nothing but being cold can present a mental challenge that is every bit as trying as the physical one (however, being experienced in meditation will help). But cold swimming in nature or in a backyard pool usually doesn't present the same level of challenge, because it is a more engaging experience that involves activity and the visual interest inherent in natural surroundings.

The practice of swimming in cold waters has a long history. Russians and Scandinavians have, for instance, been advocates of a winter splash in a river or a lake for centuries. The die-hard souls in those cultures believe the practice offers rejuvenating effects that keep a person healthy, energized, and focused (and free from the punishing effects of hangovers!).

Swimming in nature—whether it's a quick dip in an unheated swimming pool or a trip to the seaside in wintertime—offers a potentially richer experience than taking an ice bath or cold shower, as well as its own unique challenges.

Nature's Advantage

There are some advantages of cold swimming over plunging in an ice bath. The first usually involves exercise. And that's not just a matter of actually moving around as opposed to sitting still. Swimming, like shivering, produces muscle heat. That will likely result in being able to stay in the water longer than you would in a bath. It also boosts the calorie burning effect of the immersion.

There is another intangible as well. In contrast to the solitary activity of dunking yourself into a one-person tub, cold swims are most often communal activities. For starters, you need a buddy with you to be safe. But there is also a large and growing community of cold swimming clubs and

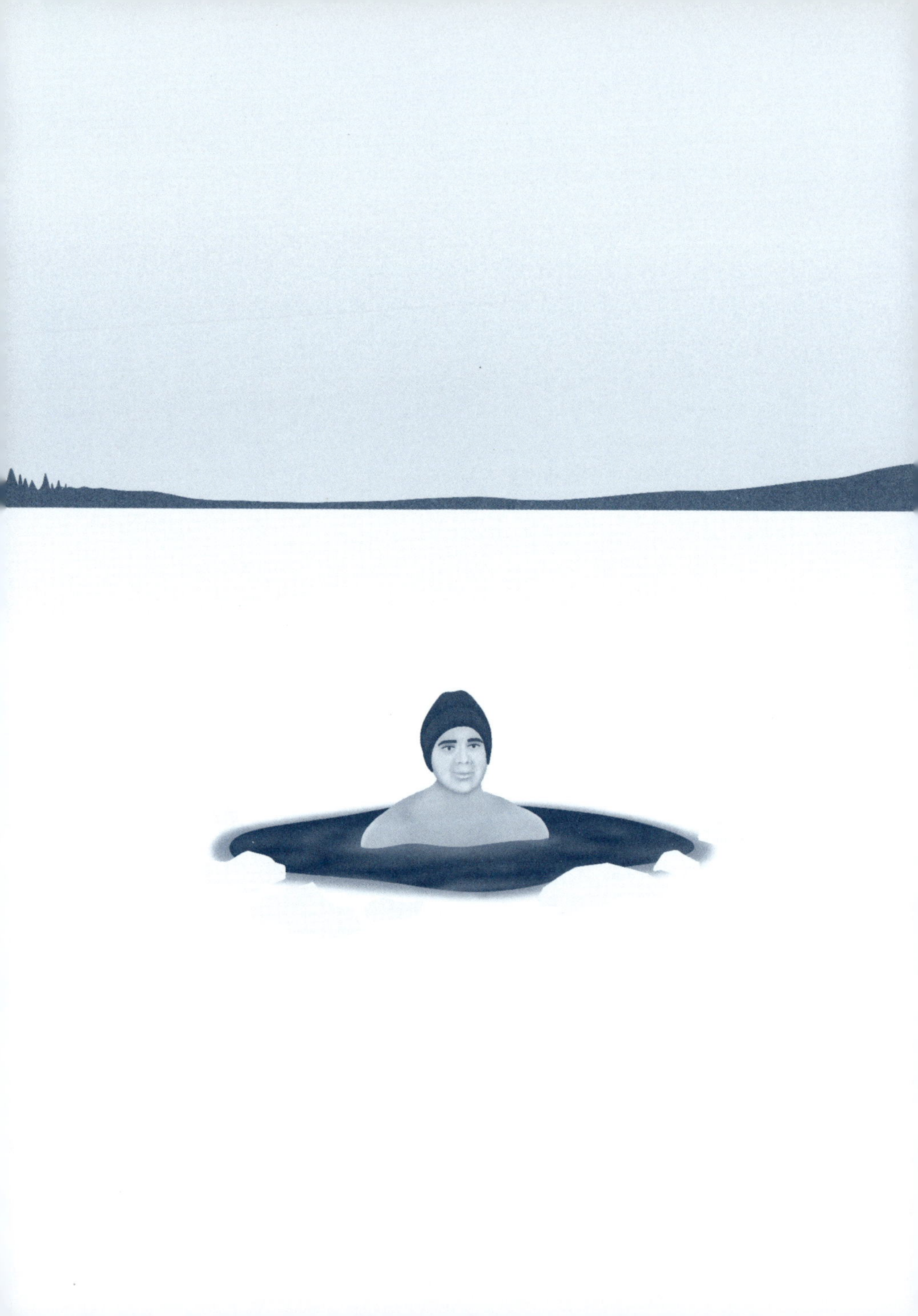

informal groups. These people share an intense experience, which leads to social bonding. Given that social interaction has been shown in abundant research to play a critical role in lifelong health, this is just one more way cold swimming may aid in ongoing well-being and longevity.

Nature's Risk

Whether you're taking a cold swim in a local pool or indulging in the wilder climes of a river, lake, or ocean, the risk is exponentially higher than it would be in an ice bath or cold shower. The depth of both a swimming pool and a natural body of water can be unpredictably varied. Given that it's preferable to avoid immersing your face or head (more on that in Step 4), uncertain terrain underfoot can lead to an unpleasant and session-ending dunk. Natural bodies of water have the added variable of other creatures who call the water home. Some may not take kindly to visitors. Not to mention, you may need to navigate aquatic plant life.

Know your environment. Even before you get into the water, you'll be immersed in cold air, often with chilly sand or rocks underfoot. This means that cold swimming requires a greater focus on avoiding hypothermia and staying safe. It also requires more mental steel.

You should never take a cold swim alone. One of the symptoms of the onset of hyperthermia is confusion. Spend too long in the water, and it is far too easy to become disoriented, forget where your car is parked, or simply lose track of how long you have been in the water.

A cold swim requires more planning than a plunge bath. It requires some additional research and prep: What is the actual temperature of the water? (You should have a precise way of measuring that, and understand that the temperature may vary in different parts of a natural body of water.) How will you quickly and efficiently heat up afterward? What routine should you follow to ensure against frostbite or hypothermia? What is the weather doing, and should that concern you enough to delay or postpone the swim? All of these factors and more must be taken into account to safely get the most out of any cold swim.

A BREATH OF (COLD) AIR

Cold water sucks heat from the body far quicker than cold air does. That basic scientific fact lies at the heart of the most recent and advanced cold therapy option: cold therapy cryochambers. These chambers enclose you in much lower temperatures for longer than you would be able to endure in water. That potentially means the benefits may be amplified. A 2000 study found that decreasing the water temperature to which a body was exposed from 68°F (20°C) to 57°F (14°C) increased the release of noradrenaline 530 percent. The same principle will hold true in a cool air environment. (Note the generally accepted ideal range for cold therapy involving cold-air exposure is a much lower -85°F to -140°F [-65°C to -96°C].)

Cryochamber technology uses either electricity or liquid nitrogen to chill the inside of the cabinet. The environment is the same in almost all models of cryochamber. The differences are expense, comfort, and efficiency.

Theoretically, you could simply expose yourself to cold air by spending time outside on a cold day while inappropriately dressed. There are two problems with that easier option: Seasons change and the weather warms, and temperatures outside are subject to quick and severe swings. It is an incredibly imprecise and hard-to-control experience. Not to mention, pretty darn uncomfortable.

Cold air cryochambers take the guesswork out of the exposure. They can be set to precise temperatures, and most are well-outfitted to make you as comfortable as possible during your cold therapy. And the procedure usually involves taking steps to protect the body's most vulnerable areas (see the discussion of glabrous tissue on page 23).

TWO CHAMBERS, SAME AIR

There are two basic types of cryochamber. The first—and the largest—is the whole-body booth similar to a sauna (they are sometimes referred to as *cold saunas*) that you step into and either sit or stand completely contained within the unit. Some even have an antechamber or "pre chamber" where you are slowly chilled, adjusting your body in preparation to enter

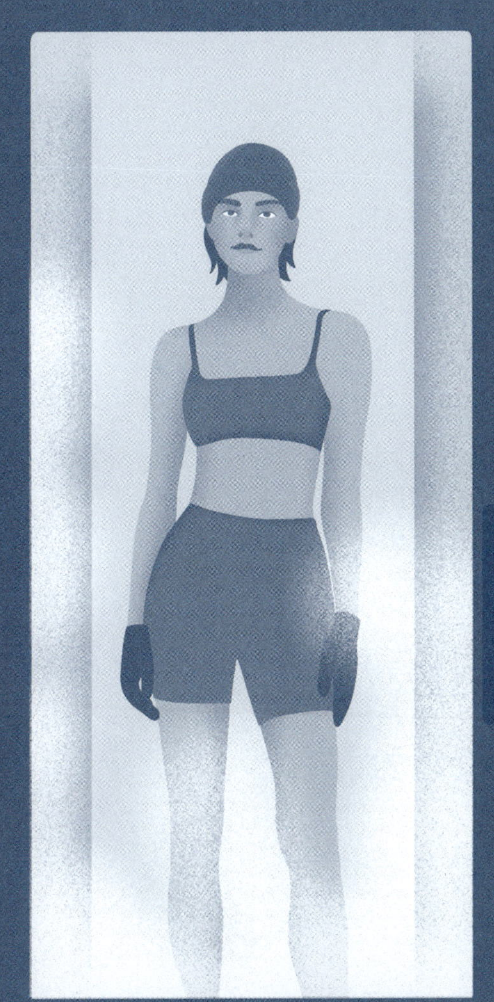
-140F

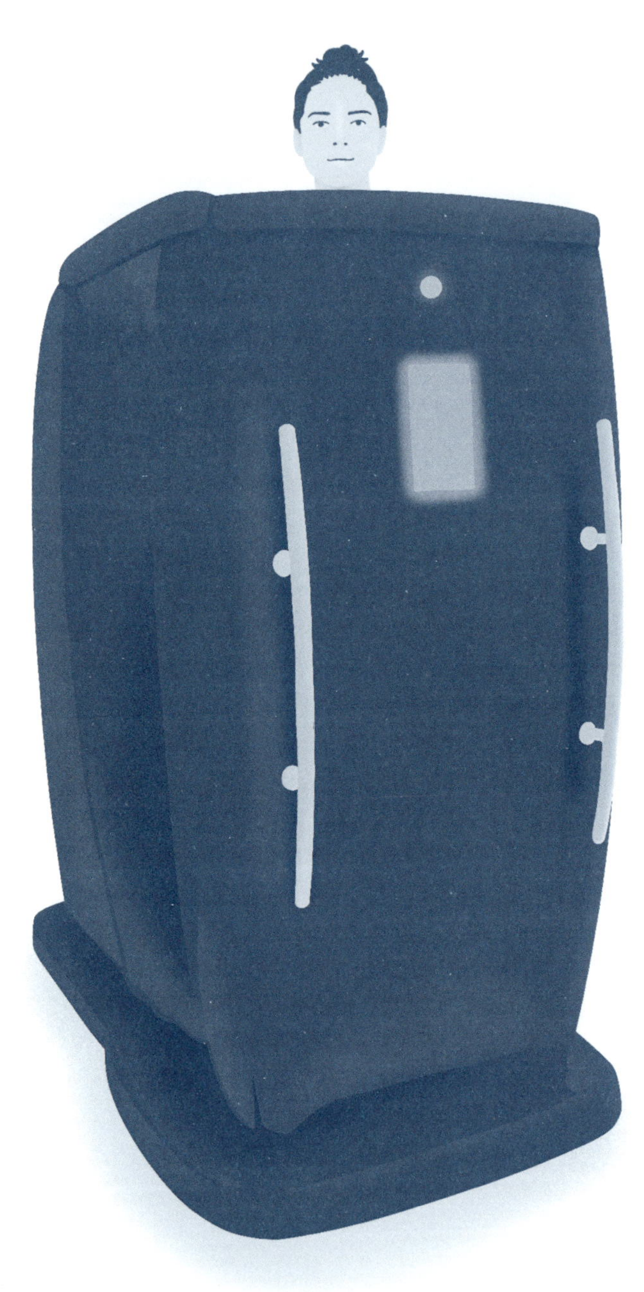

the main chamber, which is set to the low target temperature. Although many styles don't include seating (full exposure requires air circulating around the entire body), they are usually sleek in construction, with glass doors, smooth cleanable surfaces, and high-tech mechanics.

The second—and smaller—type enclose the whole body but leave the head outside; these chambers are commonly shaped like cylinders and prevent you from moving. Although smaller, these too are technologically advanced, offering options such as a screen that can stream video and monitors that track the temperature of the unit and your vital signs. Both types circulate frigid air around your body.

The industry formally refers to the full-body units as "cryochambers." The smaller sit-in models are often called "cryosaunas" by manufacturers, users, and experts. A cryosauna is essentially an oversize chair with an enclosure around it that opens and closes around you. You sit in the chamber with only your head outside.

Because the exposure is generally longer than it would be in water, cryochamber users typically wear head and face coverings, gloves, and slippers in addition to their underwear or bathing suit. Those garments ensure against frostbite that might occur due to the faster heat loss through your palms, soles of your feet, and face (see sidebar on Glabrous Tissue in Step 1, page 23).

Both types of chamber involve sophisticated technology—the kind of gear that doesn't come cheap. Few people—even staunch advocates—have the means or inclination to pay for their very own fully featured cryochamber. It's usually just as convenient—and far easier on the wallet—to use one at a high-end gym, clinic, or spa.

The temperatures are much lower and the exposure times much longer than with whole-body cold-water immersion. That means that a cryochamber could feasibly provide more powerful benefits than a plunge bath or even a cold swim could. And while there isn't as much research data available regarding controlled cold-air exposure as there is on cold-water immersion, this much is certain: It's a different type of cold therapy practiced in a different way, but to the same ends.

As you've no doubt discovered by now, you're faced with an embarrassment of riches when it comes to cold therapy options. Even if some aren't available to you—perhaps there is no swimming pool or natural body of water close enough to be a practical alternative—there are abundant alternatives you can consider.

With all of the above information in hand, you can now match the type of cold therapy that seems most promising to the health and wellness goals you set out in Step 2. Then, in Step 4, we'll create a commonsense plan of action that will help you reach those goals.

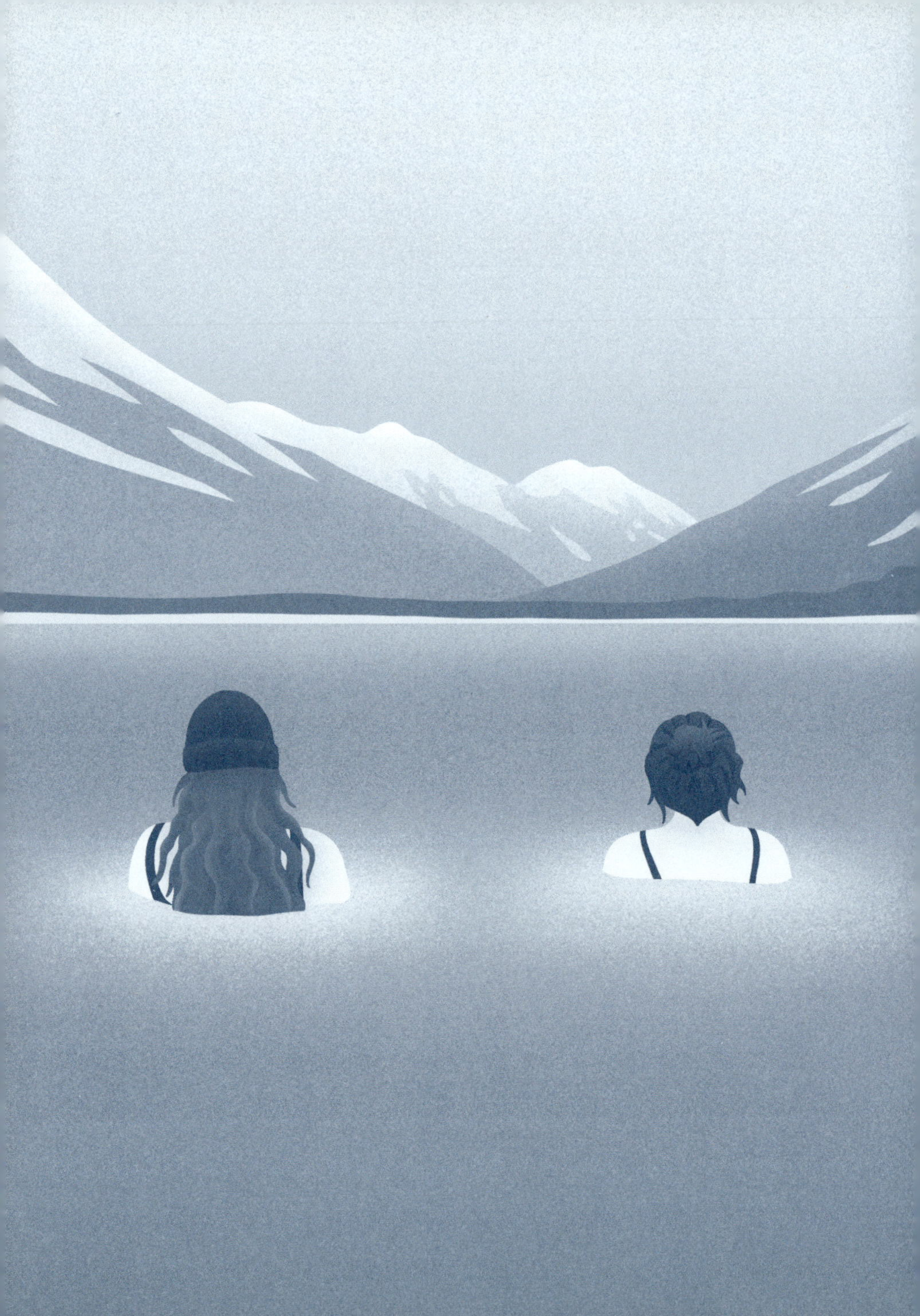

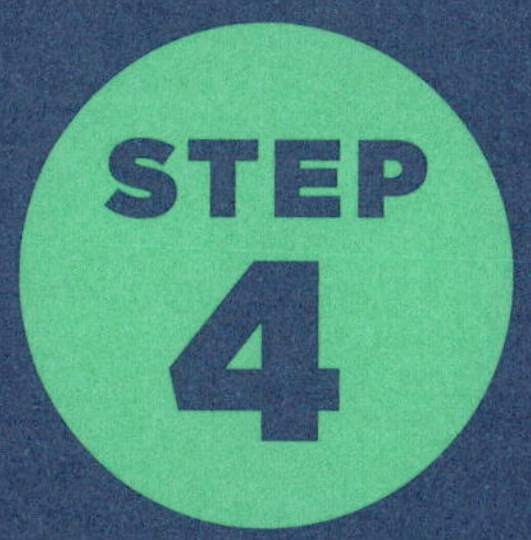

CHILL OUT

"Nothing burns like the cold.
But only for a while."

—GEORGE R.R. MARTIN

Once you've decided on a method that makes sense for you, it's time to develop your very own cold therapy regimen. It will be unique and based on your requirements and preferences. Sure, you've probably seen a lot of pictures and videos of elite athletes lounging in ice baths like it was no big thing. That's why it's all too easy to fall into the trap of thinking your cold therapy plan will be a piece of cake, something you can start at full speed and super-low temps.

Think again. Developing, sticking with, and benefiting from cold therapy is normally a matter of gradually increasing exposure. Try out what you think will work, build tolerance, and refine your regimen so that it is as tailored to you as possible. You don't answer to anyone, so approach it in a way and at a speed that is right for you. Here are the general stages you'll follow.

1. **Check your health:** The first step in crafting your own common sense cold therapy regimen is to check with your primary care provider. Your health-care professional is the expert best suited to detect red flags that might alter how, or even if, you proceed with cold therapy. Many of those warning signs won't necessarily be obvious to the individual or lay person. (See page 46 for conditions and indications that cold therapy may not be ideal for you.)

2. **Acclimate:** Most people begin their cold therapy journeys with cold showers. This is a great way to "dip your toe in the water." The experience is often easier and less jarring than jumping right into the figurative deep end of the pool with a cold plunge in an ice bath or a chilly swim in low-temperature waters. The big plus with a shower is control. You can step in and out of the spray. You can move around. It's also incredibly easy to change the spray to warmer water to gradually get used to a cold spray. (Although if your regimen consists primarily of cold showers, you should drink a hot beverage and layer up on clothing to warm up rather than finishing with a hot shower.) It's important to note, though, that showers are considered an entry step to a cold-therapy regimen, and there just aren't a lot of studies on the actual benefits of cold showers as a complete regimen unto themselves.

   Many cold-therapy advocates suggest doing thirty days of cold showers before launching a whole-body immersion or exposure regimen. That period will allow you to build up your stress response (see page 24) so that you're better prepared for an ice bath or cryochamber.

   As an alternative, you can acclimatize in a swimming pool heated to around 65°F (18°C). Immerse your body slowly, starting with feet, legs, and then the waist. This allows you to control how much of your body is exposed and for how long. Do not submerge your head.

   Although it's not an option favored by many people, you can acclimatize in cold weather by stripping down to a T-shirt and going outside during the winter months. Obviously, this is seasonal and less precise, although it does work for some individuals who live in colder parts of the world. It especially makes sense if you've settled on cold air as your medium of choice for your regimen.

3. **Escalate:** As with workout routines and fundamental changes to your diet, it's best to build from modest beginnings rather than charging in at full speed. This may entail slowly dialing up time of exposure, incrementally lowering temperature, or increasing the frequency of sessions. Keep in mind that those are three distinct variables. Change only one at a time.

4. **Tune in and fine-tune:** As your cold therapy practice evolves, pay close attention to what your body tells you. One part of your body may become sensitized to the cold or your breathing may not normalize in the particular cold therapy environment you've chosen. Being cognizant of your physical and mental state is key to maximizing any benefits you realize from cold therapy. You'll find much more detail on how to make adjustments in Step 5.

RULES OF THE COLD

It bears repeating: Exposure to cold involves risks—especially when it comes to cold water. It's essential that you approach any cold therapy with a few simple rules in mind. These ensure that your experience is beneficial rather than harmful.

1. **Buddy up:** The first and most important rule for any new cold therapy regimen is to have a buddy present. Obviously, this isn't necessary for cold showers (and that might be a little awkward). But any whole-body immersion—air or water, ice bath or lake—calls for having someone on hand in case you become disoriented or have any other unexpected reaction to the cold. Keep in mind that everyone is different in how they tolerate and process extreme low temperatures.

2. **Plan and prep:** Cold therapy isn't a fly-by-the-seat-of-your-pants type of thing. You've done your research in Step 1. Put that knowledge into action by deliberately planning a regimen. This includes establishing a target schedule and set timeframe. Decide on how you'll approach individual sessions. The more precise you are, the more likely you will be to have success.

   Detailed planning is more important when you're first starting cold therapy and aren't certain how your body will respond or in less predictable environments such as swimming in wild waters. For instance, if you've chosen to take a cold swim in a local lake during winter, it's vitally important to know how you'll strip down for the swim, dry off afterward, and warm up as quickly as possible. It's also important to measure the temperature of the water and the air. Have a plan in place if the weather turns nasty.

All that becomes much simpler if you've opted for the more controlled experience of an ice bath or cryochamber at a gym, spa, or in your home. Planning in these cases amounts to scheduling the time, familiarizing yourself with the equipment you'll use, and deciding where and how to warm up.

No matter what type of cold therapy you choose or where it takes place, mental prep plays a huge part in how positive the experience is and how effective it is in achieving your health and wellness goals. Start by setting an intention. Visualize the experience, and frame it in a positive way. It may seem silly, but this can be as basic as mentally voicing affirmations like, "This is going to be so rejuvenating!" Or, "I'm taking my first big step in healing." Approaching cold therapy with an upbeat attitude will be a surprisingly powerful tool in managing the inescapable physical discomfort that all forms of cold therapy entail.

3. **Establish temperature, duration, and frequency:** Each type of cold therapy is best developed following specific guidelines. There are a lot of factors in determining the temperature, time, and scheduling of your cold therapy. But there is one important note to consider—research has shown that the metabolic rate increases almost exponentially as temperature goes down. In other words, the lower the temperature you can endure, the more physiological benefit you'll get from the session (even if you reduce time in immersion or exposure by ten to twenty percent). Here are some specific recommendations based off of the method you choose:

   TARGETED THERAPY: This is the easiest type of cold therapy because specific instructions are usually supplied by a health-care practitioner or the manufacturer of the device you will use. Read and follow all directions to the letter, especially any safety precautions. There are far fewer risks with this type of cold therapy than there are in exposing all or most of your body to low temperatures. The trade-off is that you will not realize the whole body benefits you would from a more immersive type. Most targeted cold therapy is also intended for short-term use, such as post-surgery pain and inflammation reduction. So that means you don't have to calculate for frequency. Some forms, though, can be used to treat chronic conditions on an ongoing basis, such as knee wraps used to treat osteoarthritis.

The temperature of something like a cuff or wrap used for a chronic condition is set by the product you're using. A typical temperature is 40°F (5°C), although there may be some variation. Most units sold direct to consumers for home use do not have adjustable thermostats. Duration is another matter. A general recommendation for using a cuff to treat arthritis or autoimmune joint pain and inflammation is twenty minutes at a time for three to four days per week. If you're considering keeping the cuff, wrap, or pad on longer, be sure to check the covered skin periodically. If it begins to whiten or tingles or burns, remove the device immediately.

COLD WATER IMMERSION (CWI): The baseline of 60°F (15°C) is commonly used as a starting point for new CWI therapy, though that's not set in stone. Some people will be able to tolerate much lower temperatures from the first time they get into the water, while others may balk at even 60°F (15°C). Ice baths and plunge tubs are often kept between 50°F and 55°F (10°C and 13°C). It's a matter of balancing between registering the water as sharply cold and being able to tolerate it for the prescribed time. As you become more accustomed to the therapy, it's likely your tolerance will increase substantially. There's no harm if you feel you must start your regimen at a higher temperature than most people.

The recommended time for CWI sessions is between five and fifteen minutes, although that can vary radically depending on what your goal is and what type of cold therapy you're doing. The wide range accounts for the variation between a less predictable experience, such as a cold swim in nature, and the more precise and controlled environment of a plunge tub. In any case, be alert for any initial signs of frostbite or hypothermia—or other alarming red flags (see page 43). If you detect those, it's imperative to immediately cut the session short and recalibrate your own specifications.

Danish researcher and cold therapy expert Dr. Susanna Søberg recommends that water immersion cold therapy not total more than eleven minutes per week, with the time typically broken out between two and four sessions per week. Her research, which was conducted using young, male, cold-water swimmers as the test subjects, found that time and frequency led to the best quantifiable results.

WHOLE-BODY CRYOTHERAPY (WBC): Immersion in the cold air of WBC calls for a totally different timeframe than you would use with CWI. The air is typically many times colder than the water in the plunge tub or frigid lake. That often translates to shorter exposure times. The most common time range is from one to four minutes.

A practitioner or assistant will usually guide you through your WBC session, depending on where you go to use the cryotherapy chamber. The typical protocol includes dressing to protect sensitive areas of the body—especially the soles of the feet and hands, which cool more readily they rest of the body (see the discussion about glabrous skin on page 23). Many practitioners often wear a mask for the same reason. Many facilities supply slippers, gloves, socks and, often, a beanie or other head covering. The clothing protects against undue heat loss and tissue or nerve damage.

Acquaint yourself with the chamber and the procedure specific to the facility you're using. Some are meant for simply standing in place. Others are equipped with treadmill tracks so that you can walk during the therapy. When you're in motion, you generate heat and can often tolerate longer exposure times. Getting out of the chamber involves warming up in a prescribed process. You will likely be given a thick robe to wear. Some facilities provide a warm beverage to speed the process. You can also opt to perform light exercise to speed reheating.

Regardless of whether your medium of choice is water or air, you should be warm going in and warm up after getting out. In practice, that means undressing right before you immerse or expose yourself and warming up from the inside out by bundling up and drinking a warm beverage as soon as you get out. Note, however, that warm does not mean hot. Do not preheat your body more than room temperature before doing any kind of cold therapy.

Rewarming with a long hot shower may seem appealing, but experts warn against it. As your body works to bring core temperature back to normal, it amplifies many of the benefits of cold therapy, such as calorie burning, metabolic rate increase, and proliferation of immune system factors in the bloodstream. Quickly and thoroughly heating up your outer shell signals the body to slow down its physiological furnace, nullifying some of the positive effects. It's better to warm up slower with your normal clothes, a warm (not hot) room, and a cup of tea.

4. **Know your limits:** It's your body, your therapy, and your wellness. Go at your pace. If you find yourself hyperventilating ten or fifteen seconds into an ice bath plunge, get out. Tolerance increases even if slowly. Stick with your practice and you'll be able to build on early attempts as you increase your endurance. But if the experience is brutally unpleasant or you attempt to push your limits too far, you can put yourself in danger. An extremely unpleasant experience is also likely to lead you to abandon the practice before you realize any benefits.

TECHNIQUES THAT COMPLEMENT COLD THERAPY

There are two simple health and wellness techniques that are often intertwined with any cold therapy regimen. These help you manage the experience and can bolster the mental and physical effects of the therapy. Cold therapy advocates often use these before, during, and after cold exposure. They are also legitimate health practices all on their own. Here's an overview.

BENEFICIAL BREATHWORK

Intentionally controlled breathing is incredibly useful both in preparing for cold therapy and in managing the experience. There are many different breathwork techniques, but almost all of them aim to engage the parasympathetic "rest-and-digest" system. Because cold exposure naturally initiates the sympathetic nervous system's fight-or-flight response, breathwork can be a great counterbalance.

The simplest method is called "diaphragmatic breathing." The goal is to focus on filling and emptying the lungs slowly, steadily, and completely (something we humans are surprisingly bad at) through conscious control of the diaphragm, the large muscle that controls breathing.

The arch-shaped diaphragm sits directly under your lungs. When you breath in, the muscle clenches and contracts. It pulls down, opening the chest cavity and drawing air into the lungs. Exhale and the opposite happens: The diaphragm relaxes and returns upward into its original position, forcing air out of the lungs.

Diaphragmatic breathing is a super effective way to counteract the shallow, rapid breathing that results from cold shock. Simply focus on breathing in slowly and steadily through the nose (the nose is better suited than the throat to warm air as it flows into the lungs), purposely pushing your belly out as you do to make room for the diaphragm's expansion and allow for the lungs to inflate to their maximum. Draw air in slowly and steadily until you simply can't breathe in any more. Then slowly, and in a controlled fashion, exhale through the mouth. As you do, squeeze your core to compress the lungs and completely empty them.

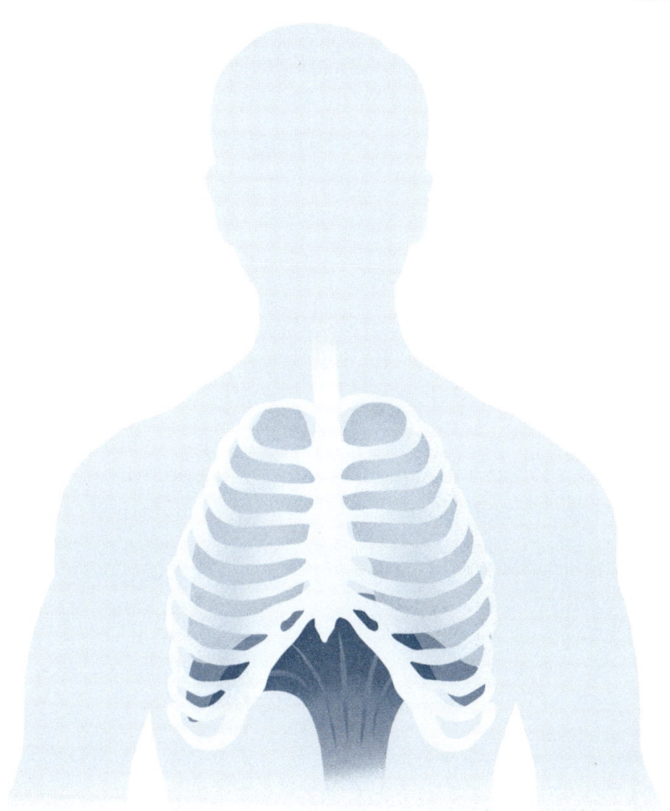

The diaphragm is larger than most people think and controls breathing, but can itself be controlled with the proper focus and practice.

This fundamental breathwork immediately slows down your breathing and allows your cardiovascular system to work more effectively in controlling the fight-or-flight reaction. Conscious breathwork floods the bloodstream with a maximum amount of oxygen, counteracting some of the disorienting effects of cold therapy. The single-minded focus on your breathing also is a great way to mitigate the intense discomfort that can be an impediment to whole-body cold therapy.

There are several types of breathwork that you can use to help you tolerate cold exposure. Most of them are effective at calming your nervous system and helping you sustain your cold therapy session to your targeted time. You can find breathwork trainers through a local holistic health practitioner, gym, or clinic, or try any of the following basic practices.

Basic Breathwork Practice 1: *Box Breath*

This breath is sometimes referred to as *four-square breathing*. It's an excellent practice for helping your body to slow down and calm down when you're experiencing stress (such as when you're really, really cold).

1. **Start with the exhale:** Exhale through the mouth while slowly counting to four, allowing all your breath to exit the body.
2. **Next, inhale:** Inhale through the nose while slowly counting to four. Feel your lungs filling completely, then feel that fullness move into and expand your belly.
3. **Pause:** At the top of the inhale, hold your breath while slowly counting to four.
4. **Return to the exhale:** Exhale through the mouth for another slow four counts. Keep all of your attention on the feel of the breath expelling from your body. Continue this breath pattern until you're ready to end your session.

Basic Breathwork Practice 2: *Pursed Lip Breath*

This practice is especially useful if you're experiencing shortness of breath, which is a common occurrence during cold therapy, especially at the start of a session.

1. **Start with the inhale:** Inhale through your nose for two counts. Don't try to force yourself to take an especially deep breath; a regular breath is fine.

2. **Exhale through pursed lips:** When you're ready to begin your exhale, purse and pucker your lips. Release the exhale through the mouth for four counts.

3. **Maintain the pattern:** After a few cycles, your breath should feel longer and more easeful. The key is to make sure the exhale is longer than the inhale, but be careful not to force or rush it. That would be more stressful!

Basic Breathwork Practice 3: *Lion's Breath*

Need to get yourself hyped up for a session? This breath might be for you. Also known as Simha Pranayama, the Lion's Breath is great for reducing stress or for energizing yourself. It can be a useful technique to help psych yourself up before taking the plunge.

1. **Turn your attention to the breath:** Notice your breath, focusing on the feel of the inhale and exhale through your nose. Allow them to be the same length.

2. **Relax the body:** Scan your body. Try to identify and release any points of tension in the shoulders, back, hips, or elsewhere. Try to cultivate a sense of relaxation.

3. **Breathe like a lion:** Take a deep, full inhale. At the top of it, open your mouth as wide as you can. Stick out your tongue, stretch the muscles in your face, and exhale, saying "haaaaaaaaaah."

4. **Continue the pattern:** Continue this cycle five to ten more times until you feel ready to start your cold therapy session. Close your mouth and return to a slow inhale and exhale through the nose to close the practice.

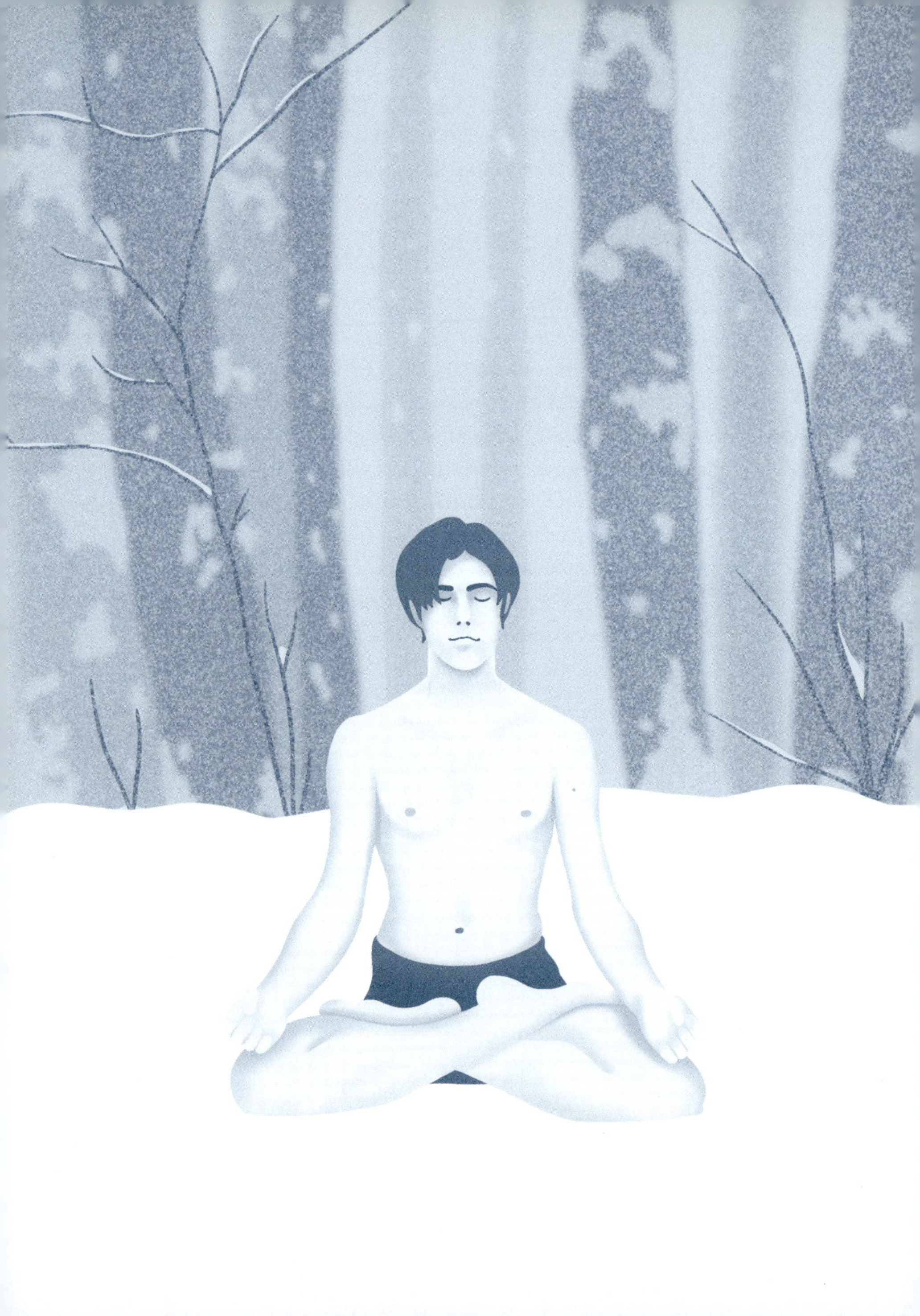

BE CHILL WITH BEING CHILL

Breathwork is not the only way to control the cold therapy process and your reaction to it. Another way to do that is through meditation. One of the biggest roadblocks to establishing a cold therapy regimen are all those panicked thoughts about how darn cold it is. Meditation is a powerful tool that you can use to minimize those thoughts and get the most out of the experience. It can also be highly effective at other times, so practicing meditation can pay off in many ways.

Meditation doesn't need to be involved or complicated. It's not some "woo-woo" practice exclusive to cave-dwelling monks or new-age types living off the grid in a yurt. In fact, as more and more people have discovered how effective the practice can be for stress relief, mental focus, and even creativity (and how pleasurable it often is), meditation has become mainstream. When used to complement cold therapy, it's an irreplaceable technique for maintaining control over the mind during cold exposure.

Start by calming yourself and clearing your mind. Choose a focal point. It can be your breath, something in your line of sight, or a mental image. Keep your attention on that focal point. As thoughts arise, just acknowledge them, label them "thoughts," and let them go. The same thoughts will arise over and over again. Don't latch onto them. Just acknowledge them, let them pass, and bring your attention back to the focal point.

It won't take long for this type of basic meditation to become ingrained as a part of your cold therapy. It will help you overcome the initial urge to get out and get warm, and it can help you reach your target time for each session. It can also amplify the mental health benefits and the simple feeling of well-being so many people realize from cold therapy.

Meditation practices can also be highly effective when used before or after a cold therapy session. Try adding one of the following practices to your regimen and see how it affects your experience.

Meditation Practice 1: *Body Scan*

Body scans are a classic meditation technique that can be used before or after a cold therapy session to witness what sensations are occurring in the body. In fact, you could even do both. It would be an excellent way to hone in on how the session affected you physically in the immediate aftermath.

The point of a body scan is to take notice of what sensations and feelings are present in the body without trying to change them, so try not to stress about what you find during the scan. These sensations will likely change from day to day and over time, especially if you're making cold therapy a regular part of your routine.

1. **Find a comfortable seat:** Allow your seat to feel really heavy, grounding into the chair or cushion. Encourage your spine to lengthen upward, lift your head toward the ceiling, rest your arms and hands where they're comfortable, and close your eyes. Allow your breath to be natural.

2. **Start with your feet:** Imagine your mental attention like a flashlight and focus that flashlight on your feet. Feel your feet and their placement on the floor or cushion, and just notice any sensations, physical or otherwise, at the level of your feet and toes.

3. **Move on to the legs:** Gently move your attention to the lower legs. Take notice of anything that arises there. Are the sensations the same on each side, or are they different? Move on to the knees, then the upper legs and thighs, noticing any physical sensation that may occur there. Also notice any feelings or emotions that may present themselves when your full attention is placed on each body part.

4. **Move on to the hips and the seat:** Feel into the general area without trying to change anything, just noticing what's present. From there, move on to the abdomen. Practice accepting whatever arises, even if it's nothing—that's fine too.

5. **Now move your attention into the rib cage and the chest:** Keep observing any and all sensations—any sense of fullness, lightness, expansiveness, limitation, movement, or vibration.

6. **Now bring your attention to the back:** Start with the lower spine and the muscles around it. Move up to the middle back, gently scanning the area for information, then move on to the upper back, witnessing any sensation that comes to mind as you rest your focus there.

7. **Move on to the arms and hands:** Start with the upper arms, then move down to the elbows, the forearms, and eventually the hands and fingers. Notice any softness or tightness, any coolness or warmth; anything that appears in the arms. Notice the position of the hands and fingers without any need to change anything.

8. **Bring your attention up to the neck and throat:** Just watch this area and stay receptive to what can be found here. Try not to judge in any way, even if a sensation is uncomfortable.

9. **Move your focus to the face now:** See the jaw and all the tiny muscles that create your facial expressions. Notice the shape and the feeling of the entire face and witness any emotions or feeling-states that may reside here. Remember, you're just watching.

10. **And now bring your attention to the top of the head:** What can you sense around the head and the top of the skull?

11. **Now draw your entire awareness outward:** Increase the size of your flashlight beam so it can witness the entire body. See if you can remain neutral to the expression of the body as it is, right now.

12. **Close your session with the breath:** Slowly draw your attention back in so that it rests in the very center of the chest and notice here the rising and falling motion that is always happening. Deepen the breath, bringing yourself back to the feeling of your body resting in the seat. When you're ready, softly open your eyes and bring your inner awareness back into the room.

Meditation Practice 2: *Color Therapy*

In this meditation, you'll use a powerful tool of the subconscious—color—to increase the power of visualization. You can choose any color you want, depending your goals and the timing of your meditation. If you're doing this before a cold therapy session, it may be helpful to choose a calming color to soothe nerves or an energizing color to psych yourself up. After a session, you may want to use a happy color to promote the feel-good vibes—whatever works for you.

1. **Prepare the body:** Find a comfortable position and allow any tension in the body to begin to soften. Close your eyes, find your breath, and begin to gradually lengthen it until the inhales and exhales are equal length. Keep breathing like this until you feel a subtle sense of calmness wash over you.

2. **Choose your color:** Now imagine a color that represents to you whatever emotional state you're trying to connect with. Take a moment and find the right color for you.

3. **Breathe your color:** As you inhale, imagine that you are breathing in this color and it is filling your body. Bright and dense, this color is flowing into you with every breath. Build the density of this hue inside the body, as you draw in the color on every inhale, and exhale just the breath back out.

4. **Continue repeating this visualization:** Keep going until your entire body contains your color. Feel it saturate your being, all of your muscles and bones, your organs, and everything from your skin inward. Stay here until everything is tinted with your color.

5. **Expand your breathing to the whole body:** Imagine you're breathing through every pore of your skin at the same time. Inhale through all of the skin, soaking in your color, and exhale out, allowing anything that feels a bit negative, fearful, anxious, sad, or uneasy to simply leave the body and dissipate. Again, inhale the color through all of the

skin, and exhale out anything you no longer need. Repeat until only that pure, calm color exists within you.

6. **Close your practice:** When this feels complete, gently guide your attention back to your natural breath. Notice how the body, mind, and emotions feel right now. When you're ready, bring the attention back to your body in the room, allow your eyes to float open softly and take a moment to enjoy this feeling. With gratitude, acknowledge the time you've taken for yourself.

Meditation Practice 3: *Immunity Boost*

If your cold therapy goals revolve around boosting immunity or promoting long-term health, this is an excellent meditation to add after a session. It might feel too "woo-woo" for some, but people used to think that way about cold therapy too!

1. **Find a comfortable position:** Lie on your back if it's comfortable or take a seat on the ground or a cushion. Bring your attention to your breath for a moment, feeling its movement in the body.
2. **Do a body scan:** Start with your feet. Take a moment and notice any sensations that are present there. Then move your attention to the ankles . . . the lower legs . . . the knees . . . Continue on slowly until you arrive at the head. Notice any feelings, any physical sensations, any information that's available in each part as you bring your full awareness to it, without judgment. If you notice any particularly uncomfortable sensations as you go along, pause momentarily and ask it to release before you move on to the next part.
3. **Begin the visualization:** Now imagine a bright white glowing light coming down through the top of the head, illuminating your brain and stimulating its connections and communication with the body's immune system—calling it to action. Let the entire skull and brain be saturated with this vibrant light.

4. **Spread the light to the rest of the body:** Envision this light traveling down from the brain into the rest of the body, filling each area up completely and seeping into every tiny space. Imagine that this light is waking up every part of the body it travels to, invigorating all of the different types of immune cells and calling upon all your protective cells to function at their highest capacity right now.

5. **Harness your army of immune cells:** Acknowledge that every cell that assists with immunity is receiving the message and beginning to circulate and search for foreign cells, or for anything that is harmful or out of place. Imagine your army of immune system cells becoming stronger—your devoted attention is fueling their training and expansion. Keep watching them as they do their work—seeking out invaders and destroying them completely.

6. **Move your focus to your entire body:** Feel your entire body now and imagine it is made up of only healthy, friendly cells—trillions of cells, full of white, glowing light and working together harmoniously. Use the power of your imagination. Let this warm glow flood over the entire body and extend out to the skin and beyond.

7. **Savor the healing:** Really try to enjoy this healing sensation that you're creating within and around you. Let the sensation of gratitude, faith, and inner trust live in your awareness. These effects will stay with you long after this meditation ends.

8. **Come back to the breath:** Very slowly, shift your attention back to the breath. Feel it moving the chest and the tummy up and down. Notice the body again resting in its seat or lying down. When you're ready, slowly open your eyes and bring your awareness back to the room.

RIGHT ON TIME

Scheduling individual cold therapy sessions is a matter of balancing science and practicality. The first decision you'll make is the time of day you'll do the therapy. Benefits can vary based on when you engage in the therapy. Obviously, timing will be dictated in part by what's most convenient for you, but it pays to know the timing that will work best for your particular goals and objectives.

MORNING

Cold therapy early in the day works best for anyone seeking to improve mental health and well-being, treat a specific disease such as fibromyalgia, address chronic conditions, and reduce pain. Cold exposure triggers all those "wake-up and feel great" mood-boosting hormones like endorphins, dopamine, norepinephrine, and others. Studies have shown that individuals afflicted with depression can be hit hardest by that disease in the morning. That makes cold therapy the perfect way to start the day for anyone wrestling with anxiety or depression. A cold water plunge early in the day also increases mental focus and can boost your energy levels for the rest of the day.

LATE AFTERNOON TO EARLY EVENING

The most significant benefit from confining your cold therapy to midday or later is sleep improvement. This occurs through multiple mechanisms: (1) the practice lowers your body temperature, which can prepare the body for sleep, (2) the final stages of cold therapy can stimulate the parasympathetic system, and (3) cold exposure suppresses the stress hormone cortisol (in fact, a 2023 study found that cortisol may be suppressed for hours after cold therapy). Both stimulating the parasympathetic system and suppressing cortisol leads to a more relaxed state, physically and mentally. In addition, the boost in mental focus helps anyone get over that all-too-common "mid-afternoon slump." All of that being said, cold therapy should not be done within four hours of bedtime. The continual effects of the therapy can continue for hours afterward and may actually impede or disrupt sleep.

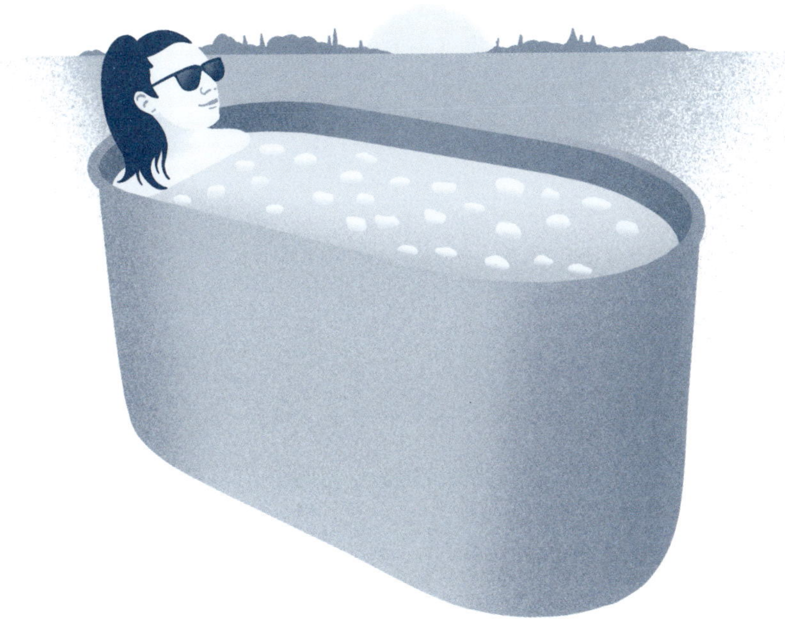

POST-WORKOUT

Cold therapy timing is most critical if you're using it to recover from athletic exertion. The sooner you get into an ice bath or cryochamber after a workout, the more effective the therapy will be at reducing muscle soreness and speeding recuperation so that you can rebound to your full competitive abilities. However, there is one exception to this recommendation. It's best to wait several hours (data suggests at least four hours) after weight training or intense resistance exercise before engaging in cold therapy, as research has shown that cold therapy can interrupt the process of rebuilding and increasing muscle mass (called *hypertrophy*).

POST-SURGERY OR INJURY

The first twenty-four to forty-eight hours are critical when dealing with trauma from severe injury or surgery. In these situations, the primary health professional will direct how, and how often, the cold therapy device is to be used on the surgery or injury site (it may involve exposure for several hours each day during the initial post-trauma period). That timing is key to alleviate pain, reduce inflammation, and speed healing. In most cases of trauma, you'll be advised to switch from cold to heat after the first few days.

As mentioned earlier, icing injuries or trauma offers short-term relief and is the best way to soothe temporary discomfort like a sprain or a tendonitis flare-up. Stick with the cold too long, though, and it can actually slow the healing process. Switch to heat to re-dilate blood vessels after the cold has done its work and reduced inflammation and pain. That process floods the injury site with nutrients and removes cellular waste products, speeding tissue repair.

DURATION

How long you should immerse yourself in any given cold therapy varies according to the type, but it is also guided by tolerance. Gradual is key in all things cold therapy. That includes temperature, frequency, and duration. A starting point is just that—only where you start. No matter what, if you continue with your practice, you will build up the amount of time you can expose yourself to cold temperatures.

The commonly repeated target limit of eleven minutes per week can seem awfully high when you're shivering through the first few seconds of your initial cold therapy session. But the idea behind building your time in exposure involves optimizing the science behind the practice. For instance, research has found that as you approach that eleven-minute mark, you significantly boost your metabolic rate and increase the conversion of white fat to beige or brown fat.

That underscores the true value of increasing duration over the course of your cold therapy regimen: You exponentially amplify the physiological benefits that any cold therapy initiates. There are also mental benefits to increasing your duration. You'll build your resistance to the stress response, which will ultimately help increase the time you can tolerate other situations involving both physical and psychological stress.

FREQUENCY

There are no hard-and-fast guidelines about how often you should schedule cold therapy, but most people find it best to allow their bodies to recover before repeating the experience. The most common frequency recommended by experts is two to three times per week. That leaves plenty of recovery time while allowing you to get enough exposure to have significant impact.

If you find it difficult to engage in the therapy as often as you would like (for instance, if a cold swim is simply not convenient more than once a week given your schedule), consider trying different types of cold therapy. This also gives you a chance to determine which is most effective in meeting your health goals. For instance, in addition to your cold swims, add in a couple of cold showers during the week.

High-level athletes, whether amateur, collegiate, or pro, usually benefit from a more frequent use of the therapy. Trainers and professionals often integrate ice baths or cryotherapy sessions five or more times a week.

However, experts recommend against overuse. There is some evidence that using cold therapy throughout a long training cycle or during the actual competitive season could possibly hamper long-term athletic adaption and muscle building. This is also true close to competition, such as the day of a game or meet, when improperly timed cold therapy could diminish peak performance.

MAKING THE MOST OF YOUR GEAR

As touched upon briefly in Step 3 (see page 78), home cold therapy devices are widely available, and many are relatively affordable. These range from small cuffs or sleeves connected to water-circulating pumps to self-contained backyard plunge baths. Regardless of what type of tech you choose, using it correctly is key to getting the most of your experience.

PORTABLE CHILLERS

At-home target-based cold therapy appliances such as wraps, sleeves, cuffs, and mats isolate the cold on a shoulder, knee, ankle, hip, or lower back. They are most commonly used for post-surgery or injury pain relief and inflammation reduction. But, realistically, anyone with a problematic joint that flares up after athletic exertion or even just at the end of a long, busy day can benefit from using one of these devices. There are many manufacturers and models available in a wide range of price points. But if you're using the device for a limited time, as in the case of surgery recovery, it's wisest to rent, which you can often do through your health-care provider. Here are the guidelines for getting the most out of one of these:

1. **Follow directions:** If the device has been prescribed by a health-care provider, follow their instructions for use. Those may differ slightly from the manufacturer's directions. If you're purchasing or renting the equipment on your own, follow the manufacturer's directions. That guidance is drafted to ensure both safety and effectiveness.
2. **Set and check:** Carefully set the unit up following the supplied instructions. Lower priced products include a water reservoir and pump and are usually filled with a half-and-half mixture of ice and water; more expensive models include a chiller and only need to be filled with water. In either case, once you've secured all the attachments, run the unit and check for leaks before starting to use the equipment.
3. **Start the therapy:** Secure the cuff, sleeve, wrap, or pad. Turn on the unit and adjust the fitting as needed. Adjust the temperature to the advised setting (if necessary and possible on the model you're using).

4. **Monitor and complete:** Regularly check your skin for any signs of irritation or cold damage. Stay relatively stationary during the therapy to ensure you don't shift the fitting. Stop immediately if you start to feel pain. Experts recommend that you not exceed thirty minutes of exposure without at least a thirty-minute break.

THE IMMERSIVE EXPERIENCE

There are many cold therapy plunge tubs and ice baths available on the market. Choosing one is a matter of balancing your budget against your needs and preferences. Because these can be expensive, it's smart to try a few sessions in a gym or other setting before committing to buying one for home use. It's even better if you have your regimen already set up so you know exactly what you need to achieve your goals. Also, keep in mind that safe practice requires having someone else nearby whenever you engage in whole-body immersion. Here's how to get the most out of a standalone plunge tub:

1. **Proper preparation:** Fill the tub with water and ice—or just water if your unit has a refrigeration feature. Set the temperature. Be precise and use a thermometer or the unit's controller for this.

2. **Ease in:** Set your timer for the session. Advocates recommend getting into the water slowly to ease the shock of the cold. This can be a mental battle, but basic breathwork can help. (See page 106 for a refresher on breathwork.)

3. **Monitor and cope:** To manage the discomfort of whole-body immersion cold therapy, focus on a pleasant visual or your breathing while still maintaining your awareness of your body. Fixating on the cold won't help you make it to your target time, but you do have to be aware of any red flags that might arise, such as dizziness or numbness in your extremities. More red flag signs of overexposure are explained on page 42.

4. **Get out and warm up:** Dry off entirely as soon as you get out of the water. Bundle yourself in layers of warm, dry clothing and sip a warm, caffeine-free beverage. It's also ideal to engage in light exercise, which can be as simple a brisk walk or jogging in place.

Cold-air immersion in a cryochamber follows roughly the same steps. However, since these units are rarely purchased for the home, it's most likely that your cryochamber cold therapy will be guided and monitored by an onsite professional. The professional will explain the process, track time and temperature, and help you warm up after your session.

UNIVERSAL THERAPY STRATEGIES

Regardless of what type of cold therapy you've chosen, a couple of simple practices will help you get the most out of your regimen (and protect against any detrimental effects).

Hydrate: As your body burns calories to replace lost heat, it also consumes moisture at an accelerated pace. That's why it's crucial to drink fluids before and after cold therapy. Water is the best, although pure fruit juices or electrolyte drinks are good as well. Although warm herbal tea is a wonderful way to slowly warm up after cold therapy, it's wise to avoid caffeinated beverages such as coffee (which can dehydrate you).

Dress for success: This applies to any whole-body cold therapy, but is typically more important when using a cryochamber than if you are immersing in water. Whether you're taking an ice bath or a cold swim, you usually need to wear nothing more than a swimsuit and a bathing cap or other head covering to avoid losing too much heat too quickly through the head. In addition to swim trunks or shorts when exposing your body to the lower temperatures of a cold air chamber, you normally wear protective footwear, gloves, head covering, and often a mask (to protect the lungs and throat lining and stop excessive heat loss through the glabrous tissue on the face).

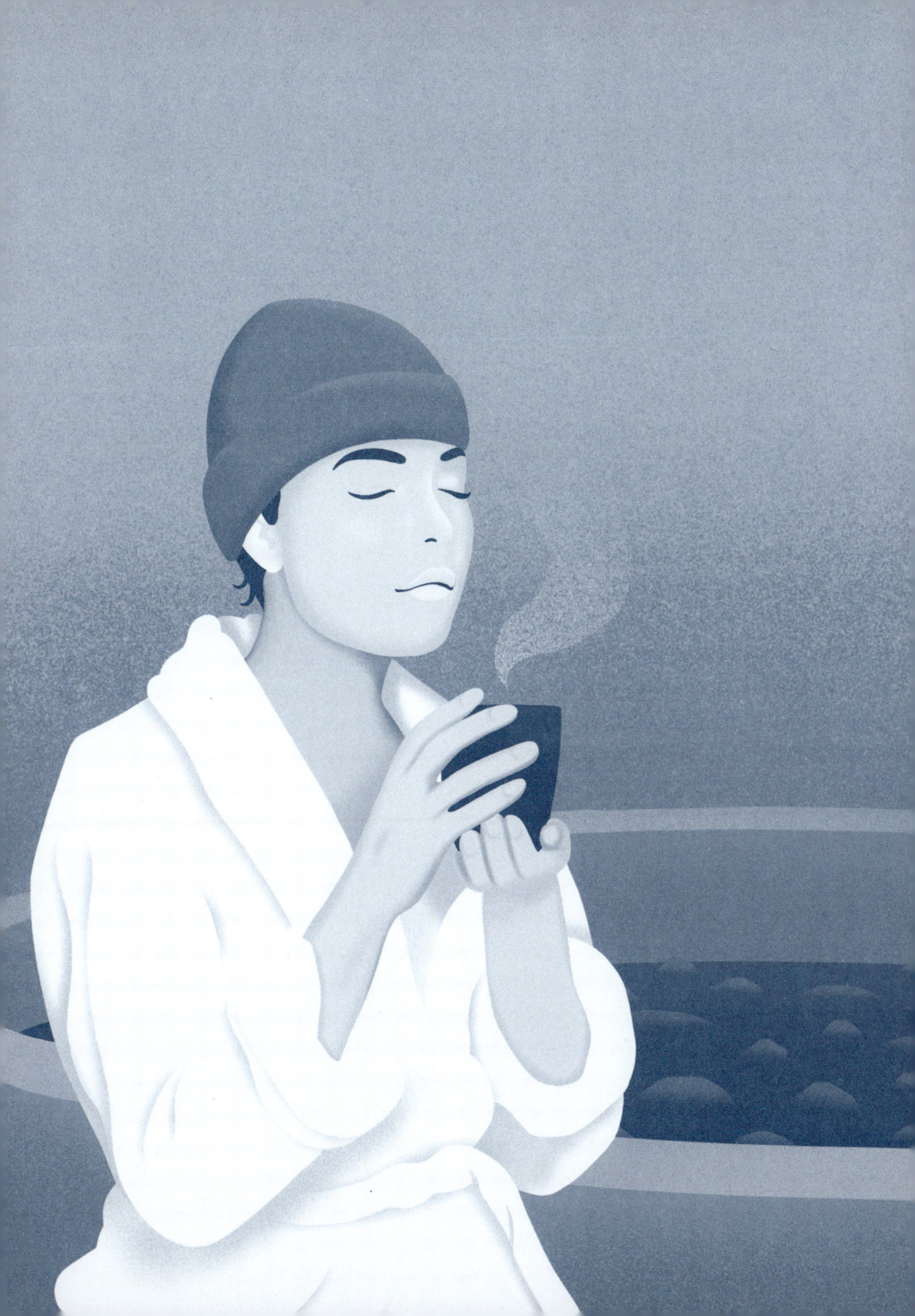

Palmar Cooling

Glabrous tissue—that skin on the palms, soles of the feet, and face—transfers heat more readily than anywhere else on the body. Although that is the reason why people entering a cryochamber are often instructed to wear mittens, booties, and a mask, it also presents an opportunity for highly effective focused cooling.

When you strategically apply cooling to your hands, feet, and face, this is called *palmar cooling*. This process has been shown in research to increase the potential work, endurance, and strength you can expend in resistance training. For example, weightlifters and other athletes use special cooling gloves mid-workout to exercise longer and more effectively.

FINAL ADVICE

No matter what cold therapy regimen you choose, always consider context. For instance, on any given day, you may be challenged by work, relationships, a car accident—whatever. Deciding to stick to your cold therapy represents a bigger challenge than usual and is an opportunity to supercharge your resistance to stressors. This can mimic the challenges (mental and physical) that you actually encounter in life and make you, for lack of a better word, tougher.

Once your cold therapy regimen is up and running, you'll likely get used to the exposure and start to see ongoing benefits. Taking your practice to the next level requires quantifying your improvement and refining the therapy to deliver exactly the benefits you need and want—and maybe even more than you expect. That's where Step 5 comes in.

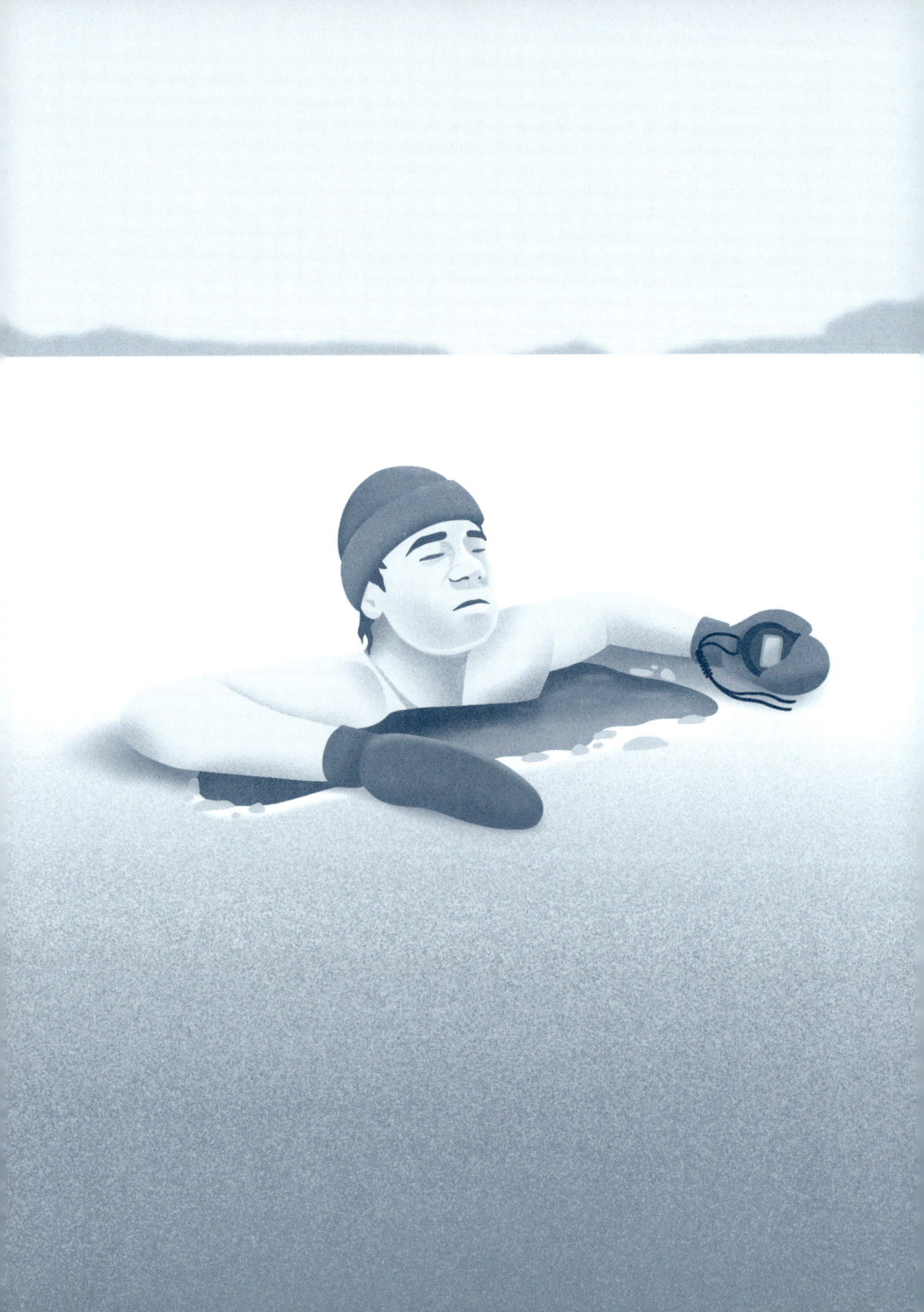

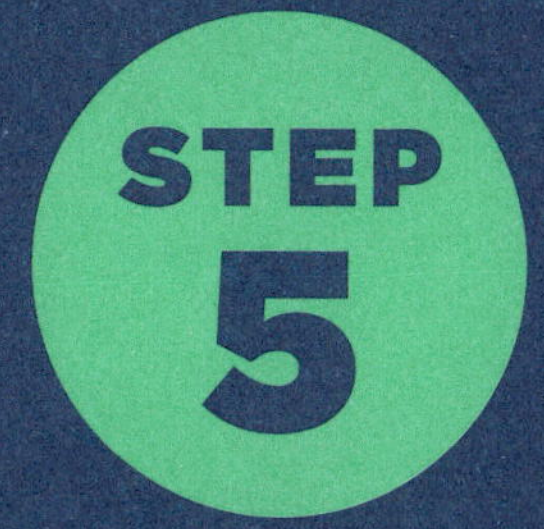

FINE-TUNE YOUR EXPERIENCE

"Winter passes and one remembers one's perseverance."

—YOKO ONO

It's next to impossible to know how effective (or not) your cold therapy is in achieving the goals you defined in Step 2 without actually noting your progress in one way or another. Because the whole point is to improve your health, wellness, and performance, you need to chart your experiences to determine if your therapy is effective—and make changes if it isn't.

When it comes to keeping track of cold therapy, everybody has their own preference. The tech-focused among us can use an app or software to digitally chronicle the history and effects of cold therapy. Some people will be more comfortable keeping a written log. You can even monitor your progress through audio or video recordings.

The point is to record your experiences and results. Chronicling the real-time progress of your regimen is invaluable for not only understanding if the therapy is having the impact you want it to have but also in giving you baselines against which you can assess, improve, and refine what you're doing. In the final step of this guide, we'll discuss taking your therapy to the next level and amplifying the benefits by making smart, data-driven adjustments.

LOG IT

Your cold therapy log should include at least the fundamental specifics about each cold therapy session. These include date, time of day, duration, and temperature, if that measure is available (and, ideally, it always should be, because you should literally know what you're getting into). Although it can be challenging to maintain a log, especially when adding more qualitative information, it helps to document how you feel before and after the therapy. Add any unusual aspects of a given session and observations about individual experiences. The more information you have to work with, the better.

ANALYZE IT

A cold therapy log is a tool. Putting it to use means asking questions that the data can answer and sifting through that data for trends that hopefully go in the right direction. That might seem a little dry, but it's essentially the same as having a doctor look at an X-ray and tell you what it means. While assessing the data, here are key questions that you might want to ask (others are certain to pop to mind):

- Can you gather enough actionable info (what researchers call a "significant sample size") before making changes or choosing to stop the therapy? In other words, have you given your therapy enough of a chance to work?
- Does the log show a valid trend that can realistically guide any plan for refinements?
- Are you realizing more of an impact from your cold therapy's duration, temperature, or frequency?

CUSTOMIZE IT

Information you can discern beyond what your log tells you will also guide how you go forward. This is where customizing your log to your own unique situation can be invaluable. For instance, if your goal is to reduce pain from a chronic condition or systemic inflammation, has your cold therapy enabled you to lower the amount of pain medication you regularly take to

SAMPLE COLD THERAPY LOG

Date	Day	Time Start	Water Temp	Duration	Type	Notes
6/1/25	Wed	10:30 am	53°F	2m 45s	Cold plunge	Barely made the time, big energy boost after
6/3/25	Fri	10:00 am	55°F	2m 35s	Cold plunge	Played music, helped with distraction from cold
6/6/25	Mon	10:30 am	53°F	2m	Cold plunge	Just couldn't do full time, felt energized
6/8/25	Wed	10:00 am	53°F	2m 30s	Cold plunge	In future have hot tea ready when I get out

Keeping track of your cold therapy doesn't need to be a burden or complicated. As this sample shows, a little basic data will give you the snapshot you need to build toward better and better results.

treat the condition? Do you take the medication less often or take a lower dose? In this example, it would be revealing to chart pain on a scale of 1 to 10 at the same time every day, as well as before and after cold therapy.

In another example, when you're using cold therapy as part of a disease treatment plan, your assessment should involve looking at medical test results. Are the numbers of a comprehensive blood panel more positive than previous blood panels? Have tests such as MRIs or CAT scans shown improvement from older results?

Or if your goal is athletic recovery, the questions may be even more basic and easy to measure. Have you increased the distance you run, your time over a set distance, your performance stats in any kind of competitive sport, or how much weight you can lift?

Lastly, what you chart doesn't necessarily have to relate directly to your goal or goals. It can be more about general health issues or the progression of your personal practice. For instance, a regular regimen of cold therapy should build tolerance, as your stress response becomes more robust. That greater resistance to stress should extend to all kinds of stress, and all areas of your life.

While you're analyzing and customizing your log, keep in mind that changes don't need to be massive to be relevant. It should be clear and apparent, though, that the numbers are trending in the right direction once you've stuck to your cold therapy regimen for a reasonable period of time—say three to four weeks.

BUILD ON YOUR PRACTICE

The data in your log tells a story, but that story is only as good as the actionable direction you take from it. Here are the basic steps to ramping up or altering your cold therapy routine to exploit the information you've gathered.

ADJUSTING THE VARIABLES

As a reminder, there are three fundamental variables to cold therapy: temperature, duration, and frequency. Think of these as dials on a stereo or other instrument. You don't haphazardly turn all the dials at once. You gradually change one, then another. The same goes with your cold therapy regimen. So let's go over them one by one:

Temperature: This is typically the first variable to tweak. Remember from Step 1 that hormone activation and other physiological changes increase as the temperature goes down and that relationship is exponential—as temperature decreases, the beneficial gains increase on a greater than one-to-one basis. However, as you lower the temperature, stay aware of your body's response. Safety is always the first consideration, and you should remain alert for signs of frostbite or hypothermia (see page 42), even if you feel much more comfortable tolerating lower and lower temperatures.

Duration: Don't be surprised if, after you lower the temperature of the water or air, you need to shorten individual sessions. Scientifically, temperature has a more powerful effect on health and wellness than duration does. If you have to slightly reduce duration to get used to a new, lower temperature, you can always look to increase the time of the cold therapy later.

Frequency: Generally, this is the variable that requires the least adjustment. That's because frequency is often determined as much by your schedule as by your goals. Two to three times per week is typical for the average person participating in whole-body cold therapy (water or air immersion). This not only fits into most people's daily lives, but it also allows a good buffer for your body to recover from cold exposure and prepare for the next session. You can still achieve measurable results with one session per week, but you'll likely notice far fewer benefits and slower progress.

For targeted therapy—if you're using a cold therapy cuff or sleeve for a chronic condition, for example—three to five times per week may be a more effective frequency to eliminate pain and inflammation. The same is true of athletes who are just beginning their training season and ramping up workouts. They can start with five sessions a week as their muscles get used to the activity. After that, they will be best served by dialing the sessions back to three to four times per week while in season or in competition.

THE ROLE OF EXERCISE

In Step 4, we covered the use of cold therapy as a recovery mechanism for exercise. But integrating exercise into cold therapy itself—immediately before, during, or right after—can add another dimension to your regimen. Exercise has the potential to boost some or all of the effects of cold therapy, depending on the exercise and when you do it. The key lies in the term "light exercise." For the purposes here, that means less than thirty minutes of moderate intensity aerobic activity. It could be a brisk walk, yoga, cycling, or similar workouts.

Adding that type of light exercise right before you start a cold water plunge or enter a cryochamber can prepare your muscles and circulatory system for the stress they're about to encounter, setting you up to tolerate

A Helpful Tweak

Refining your cold therapy regimen doesn't stop at the controls of duration and time or lifestyle practices. There is also a case to be made for "nibbling around the edges," with smaller tweaks that can still have a measurable impact.

One such refinement is to increase mental load or stress burden. Sound counterintuitive? It's actually not. This is the same thing you would do in weight training when you add weights to a bar; you are purposely further stressing your muscles to spur a response. You can do the same in cold therapy by engaging in mental exercises during a session. Although it might sound a bit odd, it's basic science. You'll strengthen the neurological pathways by working through math problems or giving yourself memory challenges such as naming state capitals or reciting songs or poems you previously learned. This is one more way to make the most out of your time in the cold (and distract from the ever-present discomfort).

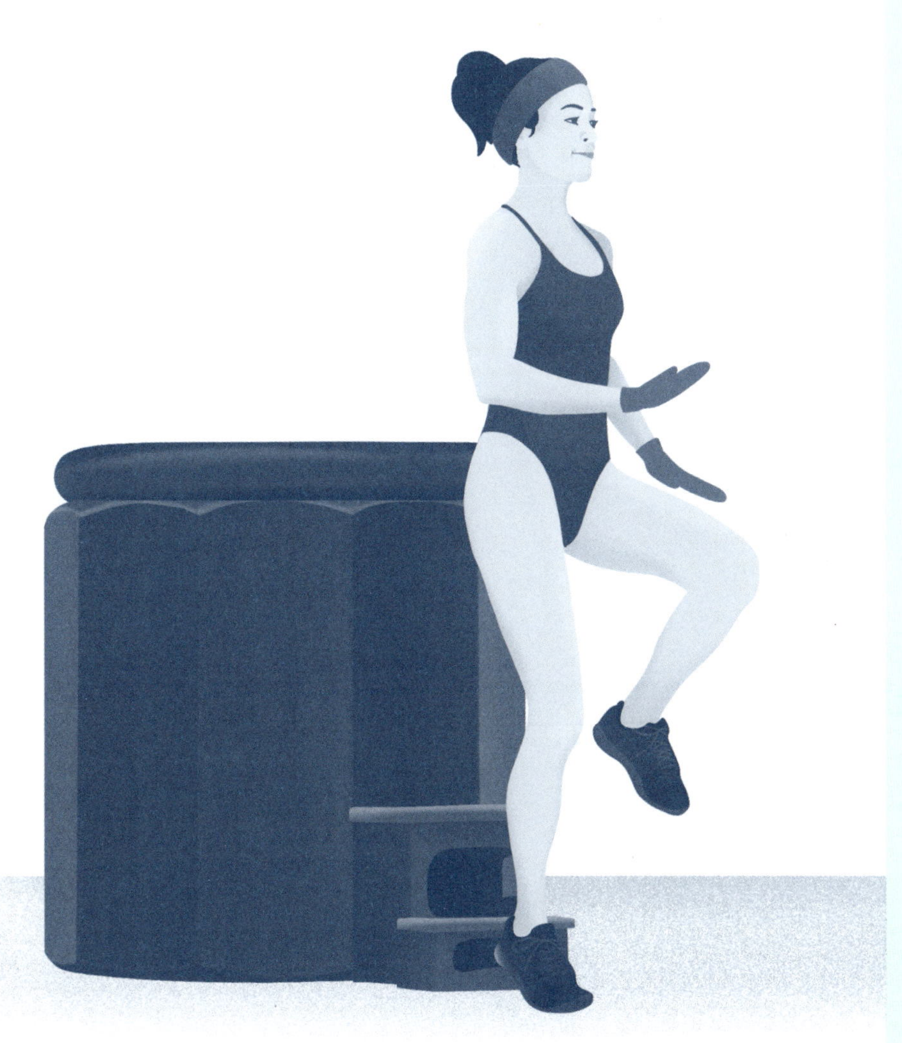

longer exposure. That said, this is the least common way to combine exercise with cold therapy.

Exercising during a session is preferable. It physically creates body heat, combatting hypothermia and allowing you to tolerate the low temperature longer. Activity in the water or in a cryochamber also keeps you occupied and makes it mentally easier to tolerate the exposure. You'll feel warmer, and the time will pass more quickly. This is why cold swimming has become so popular and why many cryochambers include an internal treadmill.

Exercising right after cold therapy can also be beneficial, if it's realistic. If you've just come from a significant period in extremely cold water, your physical coordination may be compromised enough that even a brisk walk can be difficult. But if it's a possibility, light exercise can be a safe and effective way to return your core temperature to normal more quickly than it would on its own. It can also extend the dopamine and endorphin "high" that many cold-therapy advocates experience.

A STUDY IN CONTRASTS

Another way to supercharge the benefits of cold therapy is to practice contrast therapy. A natural extension of any cold therapy regimen, *contrast therapy* is the practice of alternating extremes of hot and cold in succession. There is a long tradition behind contrast therapy. For hundreds of years, Scandinavians have done it informally. They often follow a lengthy sit in the sauna with a quick dip in ice-cold water. Advocates praise the combination as rejuvenating and invigorating. The science appears to back that up.

There is clinical evidence that contrast therapy helps maintain skin health and can improve immune system function. Rapidly expanding and contracting surface blood vessels quickly and efficiently clears cellular waste materials from the body. In fact, a 1999 study found that simply preheating before cold therapy can amplify the beneficial immune system response. That means it's reasonable to believe contrast therapy could play a part in disease prevention and general well-being, as well as longevity.

Research has also shown the potential for the practice to improve brain health and cognitive function, something that becomes even more

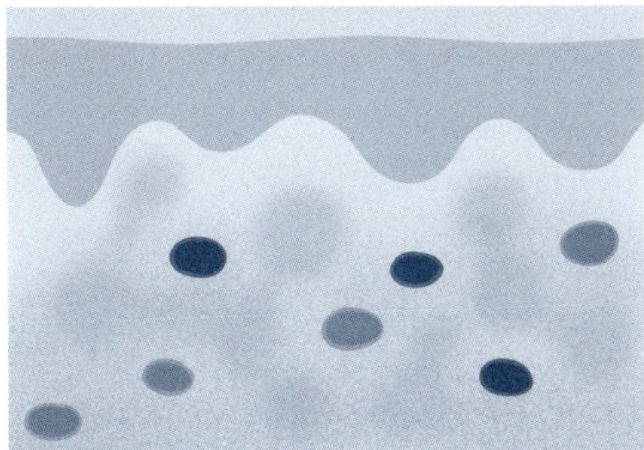

Inflamed Tissue

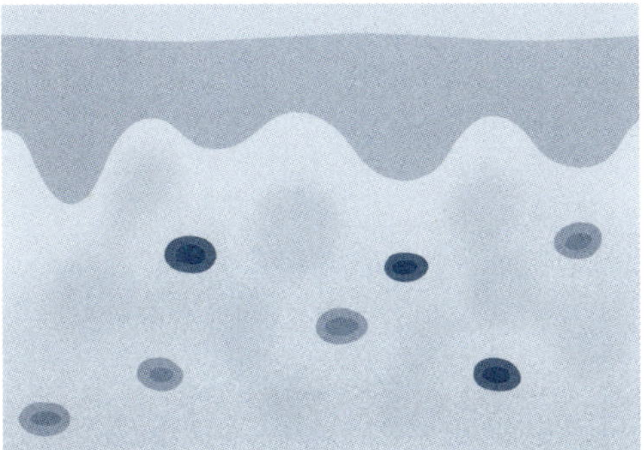

COLD
Pain signals muted; anti-inflammatory molecules flood the tissue; will ultimately aid in flushing cell waste

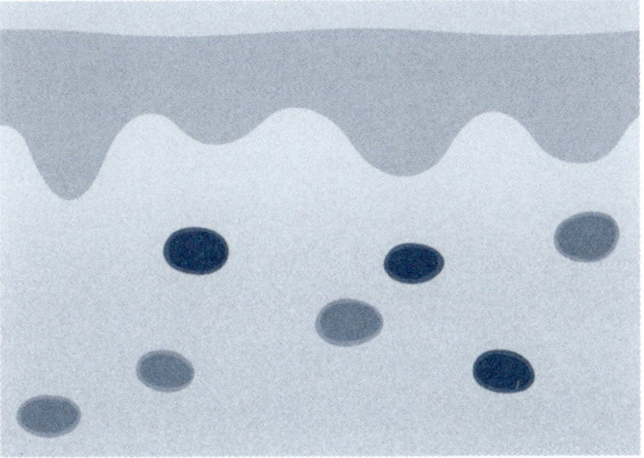

HOT
Increase in circulation delivers helpful hormones and carries away waste products from cells

important and relevant as we age. A 2015 study determined that regular sauna sessions correlated to a lower risk of neurodegenerative diseases such as Alzheimer's. The researchers credited improved circulation and a consequent flood of beneficial proteins. Alternating whole-body hot and cold exposure is clearly linked to improved blood flow to the brain. That translates to improved mental focus.

Before expanding your regimen to include hot temperatures, it's worth noting this caveat: Just as cold therapy is not recommended for anyone with heart disease or circulatory issues, contrast therapy is particularly unsuited for individuals with cardiopulmonary disease.

That warning aside, you can integrate contrast therapy for a more comfortable experience than what you'd experience with cold therapy alone. Once the body is heated, exposing yourself to a cold bath or cold air will feel far less cold than you would if you exposed yourself to cold extremes with no preparation.

Although you'll want to tailor it to your own existing cold therapy regimen, here is the basic contrast therapy process:

1. **Start warm:** Begin by spending from ten to thirty minutes exposed to hot water or hot air. This dilates the vessels in the skin and floods tissues throughout the body with blood. That action supplies muscle and tissue with beneficial hormones, protective molecules, and a host of nutrients.

2. **Cycle cold:** Immerse yourself in cold for a short time, until you begin to really feel the cold. This ensures that vasoconstriction is in full swing, helping flush waste out of cells so that it can be eliminated.

3. **Repeat more than once:** The mechanisms that drive the effectiveness of contrast therapy work best when you alternate several times between the extremes of temperature. Most people find three exposures of each extreme to be optimal and offer the most benefits.

4. **Finish cold:** Always end contrast therapy with cold exposure. This forces your body to increase metabolic rate and burn calories to return the core temperature to normal.

Studies suggest that contrast therapy can be especially valuable for elite athletes (the benefits may be less pronounced for weekend warriors). The therapy works just as well as cold therapy alone in reducing soreness and inflammation; it is also better at speeding up a return to full performance capabilities. This means contrast therapy may be most valuable for athletes competing multiple days in a row with the need to rebound quickly from high-level exertion and strain.

Where diseases are concerned, it appears that straightforward cold therapy is just as effective—if not more so—than contrast therapy. However, for some sufferers, contrast therapy may be easier to tolerate than cold therapy alone.

LIFESTYLE CHANGES AND COLD THERAPY

In an ideal world, cold therapy on its own would have the power to cure disease, counteract an unhealthy lifestyle, or make you a superstar athlete. But it is actually at its best when used in combination with other health and wellness practices. Routines as basic as good sleep habits work in concert with regular cold therapy, improving overall health and wellness and making the benefits of both more pronounced. Here are a few lifestyle adjustments that complement cold therapy:

Nutrition: Cold therapy's relationship to diet is a bit tricky and complex. Regardless, research tells us that eating well can improve the body's adaptation to the stress of cold exposure. The inverse is true, as well. Eat two glazed donuts right before jumping into an ice bath, and you're diminishing the effect of the cold therapy. To start with, your metabolic process will be strained as it tries to compensate for the effects of the cold in combination with struggling to clear excess sugar from the bloodstream. The liver will fight to convert the sugar into energy as quickly as possible to heat the core, becoming overburdened and likely converting the excess sugar to white fat. Long story short: Sugary, fatty, processed breakfasts are a bad idea before heading into cold therapy.

Caffeine, on the other hand, can support the metabolic response to cold therapy. The science tells us that caffeine will enhance the dopamine production that is already boosted by exposure to the cold. Ideally, drink or eat caffeinated foods 60 to 120 minutes before your cold therapy to take advantage of this process.

Intermittent fasting will have the same effect and can be used in conjunction with caffeine to supercharge cold therapy's dopamine effect even more. (Of course, there's only so much dietary manipulation most people are willing to undergo.)

In summary, a fundamentally sound diet dominated by plants, high fiber, complex carbohydrates, and whole foods, with minimal processed foods and little or no alcohol, will be your best bet for supporting your cold therapy regimen.

Stress: As described in Step 1, cold therapy triggers the fight-or-flight sympathetic nervous system, but does not cause the release of the potentially damaging stress hormone cortisol. That unique feature of the therapy is counteracted if you are already operating under excessive amounts of stress. That's why it's wise to take time for relaxation and down time and engage in stress-reduction techniques, such as meditation, to moderate the effect of stress in your life.

Sleep: There's a circular relationship here. The more well-rested you are, the more prepared you will be—physically and mentally—to tackle the challenges of cold therapy. But research has shown that cold therapy can also improve sleep quality and duration—as long as your timing is correct. As mentioned in Step 1, do not engage in cold therapy within four hours of going to bed or sleep will be more difficult. But an afternoon cold tub plunge can potentially improve sleep onset and duration.

THE TAKEAWAY

Cold therapy of one form or another can be a lifetime health practice, which is why it's important to keep in mind that needs, goals, and tolerances change over time and with age. The temperature that you can comfortably endure for several minutes now may be unendurable ten years from now. Always stay in tune with your body.

It also helps to periodically switch things up. That's how you keep your practice interesting; it is the opportunity to discover changes that can potentially improve your experience and results. For example, just changing the day of the week or the time of day you do your cold therapy may make a world of difference. If you can, try out a totally different type of cold therapy altogether to see if it pays you greater dividends. Switch from a plunge bath to a cryochamber, for instance. By being open to changing your regimen, you keep the therapy fresh and may possibly realize greater benefits.

In any case, the five-step process outlined here should serve as a roadmap and a starting point. Always look for chances to grow your cold therapy, and you can expand on the many benefits already inherent in this intriguing health practice. No matter what, always stay cool.

RESOURCES

ColdTub ($$$$)
Horizontal and vertical cold immersion tubs.

www.coldtub.com

Hydragun ($$)
Indoor cold plunge tub.

www.hydragun.com

Ice Barrel ($$$)
Rugged, cleanable barrel cold-plunge tubs with connected chillers (no need for ice).

icebarrel.com

National Center on Health, Physical Activity, and Disability (NCHPAD)
This nonprofit has a section on their website devoted to cold therapy's usefulness in improving mental health.

www.nchpad.org/resources/cold-therapy-techniques-for-mental-health/

Plunge ($$$)
High-end cold plunge tubs and accessories.

plunge.com

Renu Therapy ($$$)
Variety of cold plunge tanks.

www.renutherapy.com

SMI Cold Therapy ($$)
An extremely diverse range of wrappable cold therapy devices for just about every part of the body, along with information on best use of cold therapy and cold therapy devices.

smicoldtherapy.net

The Pod Company ($)
Makes small, simple cold plunge tubs.

podcompany.com
(888) 693-9031

REFERENCES

STEP 1

COLD THERAPY AND BREATHING

Cristopher Siegfreid Kopplin, Louisa Rosenthal, "The Positive Effects of Combined Breathing Techniques and Cold Exposure on Perceived Stress: A Randomised Trial," *Current Psychology* (October 2022): 1-13, doi: 10.1007/s12144-022-03739-y.

COLD THERAPY AND HEALTH POTENTIAL

Didrik Espeland, Louis de Weerd, and James B. Mercer, "Health Effects of Voluntary Exposure to Cold Water–A Continuing Subject of Debate," *International Journal of Circumpolar Health* 81, 1 (September 2022): 2111789, doi.org/10.1080/22423982.2022.2111789.

COLD THERAPY AND THE VAGUS NERVE

Manuela Jungmann, Shervin Vencatachellum, Dimitri Van Ryckeghem, Claus Vogele, "Effects of Cold Stimulation on Cardiac-Vagal Activation in Healthy Participants: Randomized Controlled Trial," *JMIR Formative Research* 2, 2 (October 2018): e10257, doi: 10.2196/10257.

COLD THERAPY AND SKIN HEALTH

Francis R. Palmer, Michael Hsu, et al., "Safety and Effectiveness of Focused Cold Therapy for the Treatment of Hyperdynamic Forehead Wrinkles," *Dermatologic Surgery* 41, 2 (February 2015): 232-241, doi: 10.1097/DSS.0000000000000155.

Robert Richer, Janis Zenkner, et al., "Vagus Activation by Cold Face Test Reduces Acute Psychosocial Stress Responses," *Scientific Reports* 12, 1 (November 2022): 19270, doi: 10.1038/s41598-022-23222-9.

COLD THERAPY AND MENTAL ALERTNESS

Ala Yankouskaya, Ruth Williamson, et al., "Short-Term Head-Out Whole-Body Cold-Water Immersion Facilitates Positive Affect and Increases Interaction between Large-Scale Brain Networks," *Biology* 12, 2 (January 2023): 211, doi: 10.3390/biology12020211.

Matthew Adkins, Rebecca Cox, John Axelsson, Kenneth Wright, "Impact of Cold-Water Hand Immersion on Cognitive Performance and Sleepiness During Sleep Inertia," *Sleep* 46, 1 (May 2023): A73, doi.org/10.1093/sleep/zsad077.0163.

COLD THERAPY AND HORMONES

Wilfredo Lopez-Ojeda, and Robin A. Hurley, "Cold-Water Immersion: Neurohormesis and Possible Implications for Clinical Neurosciences," *Psychiatry Online* 36, 3 (July 2024), doi.org/10.1176/appi.neuropsych.20240053.

COLD THERAPY AND IMMUNE SYSTEM

Geert A. Buijze, Inger N. Sierevelt, et al., "The Effect of Cold Showering on Health and Work: A Randomized Controlled Trial," *PLOS One* 11, 9 (September 2016): e0161749, doi: 10.1371/journal.pone.0161749.

COLD AIR VERSUS COLD WATER

Erich Hohenauer, J. T. Costello, et al., "Cold-Water or Partial-Body Cryotherapy? Comparison of Physiological Responses and Recovery Following Muscle Damage," *Scandinavian Journal of Medicine & Science in Sports* 28, 3 (March 2018): 1252-1262, doi.org/10.1111/sms.13014.

Kane J. Hayter, Kenji Doma, Moritz Schumann, Glen B. Deakin, "The Comparison of Cold-Water Immersion and Cold Air Therapy on Maximal Cycling Performance and Recovery Markers Following Strength Exercises," *Peer J, Journal of Life & Environment* 4 (March 2016): e1841, doi: 10.7717/peerj.1841.

A BRIEF HISTORY OF COLD THERAPY

S. M. Cooper and R. P. R. Dawber, "The History of Cryosurgery," *Journal of the Royal Society of Medicine* 94, 4 (April 2001): 196-201, doi: 10.1177/014107680109400416.

COLD AS BENEFICIAL ("HORMETIC") STRESSOR

Kelli E. King, James J. McCormick, Glen P. Kenny, "The Effect of 7-Day Cold Water Acclimation on Autophagic and Apoptotic Responses in Young Males," *Advanced Biology* 9, 2 (November 2024): e2400111, doi: 10.1002/adbi.202400111.

COLD THERAPY AND BROWN FAT ACTIVATION

Chuanyi Huo, Zikai Song, et al., "Effect of Acute Cold Exposure on Energy Metabolism and Activity of Brown Adipose Tissue in Humans: A Systematic Review and Meta-Analysis," *Frontiers in Physiology* 13 (June 2022): 917084, doi: 10.3389/fphys.2022.917084.

Susanna Søberg, Johan Lofgren, et al., "Altered Brown Fat Thermoregulation and Enhanced Cold-Induced Thermogenesis in Young, Healthy, Winter-Swimming Men," *Cell Reports Medicine* 11, 2 (October 2021): 100408, doi: 10.1016/j.xcrm.2021.100408. PMID: 34755128; PMCID: PMC8561167.

STEP 2

TRAUMA HEALING

Selman Emiroglu, Evin Esen, Nesli Yalcin, et al., "Effect of Cold Therapy on Managing Postoperative Pain Following Breast Conserving Surgery," *Pain Management Nursing* 24, 4 (August 2024): 452-455, doi: 10.1016/j.pmn.2023.03.001.

ATHLETIC RECOVERY

Feiyan Xiao, Anastasiia V. Kabachkova, et al., "Effects of Cold Water Immersion After Exercise on Fatigue Recovery and Exercise Performance—Meta Analysis," *Frontiers in Physiology* 14 (January 2023): 1006512, doi: 10.3389/fphys.2023.1006512.

Chaoyi Qu, Zhaozhao Wu, et al., "Cryotherapy Models and Timing Sequence Recovery of Exercise-Induced Muscle Damage in Middle- and Long-Distance Runners," *Journal of Athletic Training* 55, 4 (April 2020): 329-335, doi: 10.4085/1062-6050-529-18.

PRECOOLING FOR ATHLETIC PERFORMANCE

Maria Roriz, Pedro Brito, et al., "Performance Effects of Internal Pre- and Pre-Cooling Across Different Exercise and Environmental Conditions: A Systematic Review," *Frontiers in Nutrition* 9 (October 2022): 959516, doi: 10.3389/fnut.2022.959516.

Paul R. Jones, Christian Barton, Dylan Morrissey, et al., "Pre-Cooling for Endurance Exercise Performance in the Heat: A Systematic Review," *BMC Medicine* 10, 166 (March 2012): doi.org/10.1186/1741-7015-10-166.

CANCER TREATMENT (CRYOIMMUNOTHERAPY)

Tatiana P. Grazioso, Nabil Djouder, "The Forgotten Art of Cold Therapeutic Properties in Cancer: A Comprehensive Historical Guide," *iScience* 26, 7 (July 2023): 107010, doi.org/10.1016/j.isci.2023.10701.

FIGHTING AUTOIMMUNE DISEASE PAIN

Martina Spiljar, Karin Steinbach, et al., "Cold Exposure Protects from Neuroinflammation Through Immunologic Reprogramming," *Cell Metabolism* 33, 11 (November 2021): 2231-2246, doi: 10.1016/j.cmet.2021.10.002.

DIABETES AND BLOOD SUGAR

Yoanna M. Ivanova, Denis P. Blondin, "Examining the Benefits of Cold Exposure as a Therapeutic Strategy for Obesity and Type 2 Diabetes," *Journal of Applied Physiology* 130, 5 (May 2021): 1448-1459, doi: 10.1152/japplphysiol.00934.2020.

IMPROVING IMMUNE SYSTEM RESPONSE

Ladislav Jansky, D. Tereza Pospisilova, et al., "Immune System of Cold-Exposed and Cold-Adapted Humans," *European Journal of Applied Physiology and Occupation Physiology* 72, 5-6 (1996): 445-450, doi: 10.1007/BF00242274.

W. G. Siems, R. Brenke, et al., "Improved Antioxidative Protection in Winter Swimmers," *QJM: An International Journal of Medicine* 92, 4 (April 1999): 193-198, doi.org/10.1093/qjmed/92.4.193.

MENTAL HEALTH

Nokolai A. Shevchuk, "Adapted Cold Shower as a Potential Treatment for Depression," *Medical Hypotheses* 70, 5 (November 2008): 995-1001, doi: 10.1016/j.mehy.2007.04.052.

John S. Kelly, Ellis Bird, "Improved Mood Following a Single Immersion in Cold Water," *Lifestyle Medicine* 3, 1 (January 2022): e53, doi.org/10.1002/lim2.53.

Christoffer van Tulleken, Michael Tipton, et al., "Open Water Swimming as a Treatment for Major Depressive Disorder," *BMJ Case Reports* (August 2018): bcr2018225007, doi: 10.1136/bcr-2018-225007.

Nikolai A. Shevchuk, "Adapted Cold Shower as a Potential Treatment for Depression," *Medical Hypotheses* 70, 5 (2008): 995-1001, doi: 10.1016/j.mehy.2007.04.052.

POTENTIAL WEIGHT LOSS (THERMOGENESIS AND BROWN FAT)

Anouk A. J. J. van der Lans, Joris Hoeks, et al., "Cold Acclimation Recruits Human Brown Fat and Increases Nonshivering Thermogenesis," *The Journal of Clinical Investigation* 123, 8 (July 2013): 3395-3403, doi: 10.1172/JCI68993.

SKIN HEALTH AND APPEARANCE

Francis R. Palmer, Michael Hsu, et al., "Safety and Effectiveness of Focused Cold Therapy for the Treatment of Hyperdynamic Forehead Wrinkles." *Dermatologic Surgery* 41, 2 (February 2015): 232-241, doi: 10.1097/DSS.0000000000000155.

STEP 3

COLD SHOWERS AND IMMUNE RESPONSE

Mahmoud R. M. El-Ansary, Amira R. El-Ansary, Sereen M. Said, Mohamed A. Abdel-Hakeem, "Regular Cold Shower Exposure Modulates Humoral and Cell-Mediated Immunity in Healthy Individuals," *Journal of Thermal Biology* 125 (October 2024): 103971, doi.org/10.1016/j.jtherbio.2024.103971.

RELEVANCE OF WATER TEMPERATURE

Petr Sramak, Marie Simeckova, et al., "Human Physiological Responses to Immersion into Water of Different Temperatures," *European Journal of Applied Physiology* 81 (February 2000): 436-442, doi.org/10.1007/s004210050065.

STEP 4

CORTISOL AND SLEEP

Emma L. Reed, Christopher L. Chapman, et al., "Cardiovascular and Mood Responses to an Acute Bout of Cold Water Immersion," *Journal of Thermal Biology* 118 (December 2023): 103727, doi: 10.1016/j.jtherbio.2023.103727.

STEP 5

CONTRAST THERAPY

I. K. M. Brenner, J. W. Castellani, et al., "Immune Changes in Humans During Cold Exposure: Effects of Prior Heating and Exercise," *Journal of Applied Physiology* 87, 2 (August 1999): 699-710, doi.org/10.1152/jappl.1999.87.2.699.

Tanjaniina Laukkanen, Hassan Khan, et al., "Association Between Sauna Bathing and Fatal Cardiovascular and All-Cause Mortality Events," *JAMA Internal Medicine* 175, 4 (April 2015): 542-548, doi:10.1001/jamainternmed.2014.8187.

Francois Bieuzen, Chris M. Bleakley, Joseph Thomas Costello, "Contrast Water Therapy and Exercise Induced Muscle Damage: A Systematic Review and Meta-Analysis." *PLOS One* 8, 4 (April 2023): e62356, doi: 10.1371/journal.pone.0062356.

Marcello Solinas, Sergi Ferre, et al., "Caffeine Induces Dopamine and Glutamate Release in the Shell of the Nucleus Accumbens," *The Journal of Neuroscience* 22, 15 (August 2002): 6321-6324, doi: 10.1523/JNEUROSCI.22-15-06321.2002.

PALMAR COOLING AND ATHLETICS

Dennis A. Grahn, Vinh H. Cao, et al., "Work Volume and Strength Training Responses to Resistive Exercise Improve with Periodic Heat Extraction from the Palm," *Journal of Strength and Conditioning Research* 26, 9 (September 2012): 2558-2569, doi: 10.1519/JSC.0b013e31823f8c1a.

ABOUT THE AUTHOR

Chris Peterson is an experienced writer with more than twenty-five books to his credit, covering topics from health and cooking to memoirs. His work includes *The CBD Skincare Solution: The Power of Cannabidiol for Healthy Skin* (with Dr. Manisha Singal), *The Everyday Meat Guide* (with Ray Venezia), and *Better Than New: Lessons I've Learned from Saving Old Homes (and How They Saved Me)* (with HGTV host Nicole Curtis). Chris lives and works in the small town of Ashland, Oregon.

INDEX

D

S

T

V

W